TIME TO SAVE MEDICINE

Abhijit Naskar is the twenty-first century mind of science, whose glorious philosophical touch has enabled modern Neuroscience to effectively engage in the human society towards diminishing the ever-growing conflicts among religions. As an untiring advocate of global harmony and peace, he became a beloved best-selling author all over the world with his very first book "The Art of Neuroscience in Everything". With various of his pioneering ventures into the Neuropsychology of religious sentiments, he has hugely contributed to humanity's attempt of eradicating religious differences, for which he is popularly hailed as a humanitarian who incessantly works towards taking the human civilization in the path of sweet general harmony.

TIME TO SAVE
MEDICINE

ABHIJIT NASKAR

Time to Save Medicine

Copyright © 2018 Abhijit Naskar

This is a work of non-fiction

All rights reserved. No part of this publication may be reproduced, distributed, or transmitted in any form or by any means, including photocopying, recording, or other electronic or mechanical methods, without the prior written permission of the author, except in the case of brief quotations embodied in critical reviews and certain other noncommercial uses permitted by copyright law.

An Amazon Publishing Company, 1st Edition, 2018

Printed in United States of America

ISBN: 9781724111562

Also by Abhijit Naskar

The Art of Neuroscience in Everything
Your Own Neuron: A Tour of Your Psychic Brain
The God Parasite: Revelation of Neuroscience
The Spirituality Engine
Love Sutra: The Neuroscientific Manual of Love
Homo: A Brief History of Consciousness
Neurosutra: The Abhijit Naskar Collection
Autobiography of God: Biopsy of A Cognitive Reality
Biopsy of Religions: Neuroanalysis towards Universal Tolerance
Prescription: Treating India's Soul
What is Mind?
In Search of Divinity: Journey to The Kingdom of Conscience
Love, God & Neurons: Memoir of a scientist who found himself by getting lost
The Islamophobic Civilization: Voyage of Acceptance
Neurons of Jesus: Mind of A Teacher, Spouse & Thinker
Neurons, Oxygen & Nanak
The Education Decree
Principia Humanitas
The Krishna Cancer
Rowdy Buddha: The First Sapiens
We Are All Black: A Treatise on Racism
The Bengal Tigress: A Treatise on Gender Equality
Either Civilized or Phobic: A Treatise on Homosexuality
Wise Mating: A Treatise on Monogamy
Illusion of Religion: A Treatise on Religious Fundamentalism
The Film Testament
Human Making is Our Mission: A Treatise on Parenting
I Am The Thread: My Mission
7 Billion Gods: Humans Above All
Lord is My Sheep: Gospel of Human
Morality Absolute
A Push in Perception
Let The Poor Be Your God
Conscience over Nonsense
Saint of The Sapiens

DEDICATION

Hunter Doherty "Patch" Adams
Mother Teresa

CONTENTS

You are The Medicine 1
Bibliography 77

You are The Medicine

ABHIJIT NASKAR

Medicine is not merely a field of scientific knowledge - it is a backup force of life. Medicine stands at the forefront of humankind's greatest and most magnificent achievements. And in this amazingly "magnastic" (I coin here the term "magnastic" as an adjective to describe "magnificent" and "fantastic" together) feat of humanity, the urge for knowledge has played a crucial role, but as far as the practice of medicine is concerned, knowledge alone is nothing but worthless piece of empirical information.

Knowledge must be born from empirical understanding surely, but it must not be bound to the limitations of empiricism, for imagination is no empiricism, yet some of the greatest wisdoms that manifested in the human universe were realized through imagination. Hence, once born, knowledge must spread its wings and make the mind comprehend even the incomprehensible.

There is a difference between medical knowledge and medical wisdom. Medical knowledge is merely the understanding of sickness and its possible treatments, whereas medical wisdom is about having a deeper insight of human wellbeing, beyond the simple understanding of sickness and treatments. With medical knowledge one may treat a sick body and make it function properly for a short period of time, but it is with medical wisdom, that one can treat a human being, suffering from a certain sickness, and have a lasting impact on the person's existence.

Medical knowledge only can postpone sickness and death, but it is in the power of medical wisdom to sustain life with all its colors, sweetness and textures. So, don't just acquire medical knowledge, work on that knowledge with the force of your conscience and turn it into the most effective medical wisdom in the history of medicine. You are not a soulless computer that acquires more and more data, without actually knowing the actual use of that data. Acquiring more and more medical data doesn't make you a good doctor, what does, is your ability to see through that data and utilize it to heal not just the patient's body, but his or her entire being.

There is a difference between a doctor of humans and a mechanic of machines. A mechanic fixes machines, whereas a doctor restores the spirit in humans. You are a doctor, not a mechanic. So, act like one. However, more and more so-called doctors of today are trained as mechanics who fix the human body instead of trying to heal the human being. But, don't let the psyche of majority fool you – expand your consciousness beyond the size of your society. A land of mechanics may try its best to turn you into a mechanic, but forget not, that you are a doctor who heals, not a mechanic who fixes.

Practice of Medicine is unlike most other scientific practices, where the love of one's field, makes the person a good practitioner of that field. Love of Mathematics, makes a person a good mathematician, love of physics makes a person a good physicist, love of chemistry makes a person a good chemist. But when it comes to medicine, or to be specific, practice of medicine, it's not the love of medicine that makes a person a good doctor, it's the love of humanity. Love of medicine may make you a good medical researcher, but not a good medical doctor.

A good doctor - that's what you ought to be concerned of being - and the only way to be so, is to foster a plain, ordinary, everyday love for humanity. And if you need to make efforts to understand this very sentence and in fact to foster the love I'm talking about, then perhaps, medical practice is not your field. Because the practice of medicine is not just about you the practitioner, it's about the people the practitioner would have to deal with, day in day out. And without the basic love for humanity, this ordeal would only bring misery upon your soul - and this inpouring of misery would slowly but inadvertently outpour through your behavior upon your patients.

Here I am not asking you to be happy all the time, rather I am talking about being aware of whether your everyday encounter with the patients is turning out to be the darkest nightmare for you. Remember, denial of the self accomplishes nothing good. So, be aware at all times - be aware of your joy - be aware of your sorrows - be aware of your ambitions - be aware of your thoughts - be aware of your behavior.

Don't judge, analyze or criticize - just be aware - in the simplest manner possible. Awareness must be an effort-less act of the mind, otherwise, it's no awareness. And that awareness would automatically entail the right path for you to walk on, as an essential part of the awareness itself. In that awareness, you and the path you walk on, are not separate - they are one indivisible entity - a living ever-evolving entity, that exudes meaning into the meaningless world as it moves ahead with the force of conscience running through your veins.

In simple terms, when you are truly aware, the path begins to manifest itself through the pedestrian - through you - and you begin to walk on it without even being aware that you are actually walking on a path - because the path is not just a path anymore - it reveals itself as the very expression of your existence. When true awareness is at play, the pedestrian becomes the path and the path becomes the pedestrian - the aware becomes the awareness and awareness becomes the aware. And when this awareness manifests within you, you no longer need to ask someone else, what the right path is, for you truly, actually, genuinely become the right path yourself - you become the lifeforce of the path.

And when you walk on this path of liberation as a good, conscientious doctor, the right capacity for diagnosis materializes in your mind by itself.

You do not need to be able to diagnose a patient's condition right at sight unless you are in the OR, but you must be able to genuinely recognize and realize the worry and weakness in the patient's mind right from the very beginning. Remember, you will never be a first-class doctor until you learn to have some regard for human frailty.

Treat the body with all your medical capacity, but remember to heal the mind as well, because without a healthy mind, even the healthiest body turns sick. Not every sickness is psychosomatic, but a weak psyche can indeed make a sickness worse. So, don't just focus on treating the physiology, but treat the physiology and psychology together, for they are intertwined in sickness and in health. And this is only possible when your practice is predicated on kindness and not on economic benefit.

A tiny gesture of kindness can improve the brain-health of the patient exponentially, which would in turn improve bodily-health. This process begins with the building of a patient-doctor bond of trust through the release of a neurochemical called oxytocin. For a patient to be fully treated by a doctor, the patient must be willing to put all psychological guards down and be vulnerable. And this can only happen if the patient can trust the doctor, and this trust can only be induced through the release of oxytocin, which can only be triggered in the patient's brain by the will of a doctor with a genuine act of kindness on the doctor's part. The higher the level of trust between a patient and a doctor, the faster the recovery. And the gesture of kindness that is the seed of this trust, manifests in your behavior quite naturally once you recognize your innate humanity.

Humanity is yet to become human, so the human must become the humanity. The human - the individual, self-aware, nondualistic and whole human being, must become the eyes and ears and voice and footsteps of the whole humanity. Humanity as a species is not humane, and humanity as a quality is not yet humane either, so, how can the term humanity be real in the first place - isn't it just a cheap imitation of what really could be humanity! Humanity without humanity is no humanity, it's only a mockery of humanity.

So, the need has finally arisen, for the humans to stand up, in order to make humanity come true, otherwise, we will end up as yet another dying species - and unlike other animal species, we will not die probably of starvation or sickness, rather we will die due to our intellectual stupidity - due to the unrealization of our innate humanity. So, time has come my friend, that you stop letting the animals around you from conditioning you with their barbarian preaching, masquerading as pompous ideologies, be it nationalist, cultural, political, religious or intellectual, and start becoming truly aware of what humanity truly is, both as a quality and as a species.

I can't expect from the non-human animals much, because they don't have the brain capacity to become much more than what they already are. But the human animals on the other hand, are a radically different story. We are not humans yet, but we can be, if we really, genuinely, actually desire to be so. We can be humans, we can be messiahs, we can be living, actual, genuine real gods on this planet. And perhaps, no other being is required to realize this simple fact of mortal life, more than you, my dear doctor.

Believe it or not, my dear indomitable doctor, you are a living messiah on this planet, hence, every word of yours matters to the patient way more than the words of any other person. So, choose your words wisely. Words can strengthen the weak, words can rejuvenate the meek - words can breathe life into the dead, words can unite the divided - words can bring smile on the face of the unfortunate, words can encourage the hearts of the desperate – words can alleviate the anguish of humanity, words can sow the seeds of serenity. Words are not merely a bunch of syllables uttered together - when brought adjacent to each other, the right combination of words can construct the real abode of peace and progress, which most humans only dream of.

Dreams are like seeds, which won't become actual fruit-bearing trees until someone stands up to sow these seeds with care. Dreaming without effort is mere waste of brain chemicals. Everyone can dream big, but not everyone becomes big, because those who become big use less of their mental potential to dream and more to make that dream a reality, whereas the ordinary masses use up almost all their mental potential to simply dream and do nothing tangible to make it a reality. Reality is a mental construct, as such it is mouldable, be it a personal reality or a social reality, but it can only be moulded by the persistent. Reality begins with realization.

Realization is the first step to creation. Then comes the requirement of courage and persistence to walk on the path that others wouldn't even dare to set foot on, for it appears to them to be too absurd and downright impossible. And absurdity of an idea is precisely the criterion of a great idea. When I quit my university, people in my neighborhood quite literally began to gossip about me being insane, while others pitied me as a lost soul.

But mark this my friend, it's the lost souls that lay the foundation for a better tomorrow, because those beings are not afraid to be lost, they are not afraid to fail, in the pursuit of something greater, something grander, than to just survive no different than the dogs do on the streets. Legends become legends by getting lost, so that humanity doesn't.

As such, I am not afraid to die, but I am afraid not to live. So, I chose to build my path - a path of liberation - a path of truth - a path of realization - a path of life beyond survival. And I didn't mind dying while trying to lay the foundation of that path which would one day unify the whole humanity beyond the primordial loyalty to images, symbols and labels.

So, build your path my friend – build that path that's unique to you. Most so-called doctors may boastfully proclaim to you that you must be concerned about making a lot of money in the practice of medicine, but keep in mind, that's precisely what practice of medicine is not about. So, reply to them with utmost realization of the purpose of medicine, "if you want to make a lot of money, then you should better go into business, not in medicine." Here, I am not talking about denying the importance of money, I am simply mentioning the real purpose of money, for once you are addicted to the urge for making more and more money, that craving would eventually possess you and turn you into a material monster from a true healer.

In today's world, money is like oxygen - lack of oxygen can kill you, so can too much of it. The same is for money, you just need enough of it to live, but not more., for in case of the ordinary mortal human, possession of more money leads to a craving for more material possession which you can buy with that money, that in turn leads to an obsession over the possession of more money. And this chain reaction keeps running, until every cell in your body begins to die of psychological dependency, as you slowly but unavoidably begin to be consumed by consumerism.

Money is not the enemy - the humans have become the enemy of themselves. The instincts that once kept them alive in the jungle have finally turned against them as they have made unimaginable progress in the external world without paying even the slightest bit of attention to internal progress. So I say, turn your eyes and ears toward yourself, and you shall naturally begin to find answers to questions for which you would have previously gone to a so-called expert. Here I am not talking about technical answers, I'm talking about everyday psychological answers related to life.

Remember, there is no predestined meaning of life, other than what you make of it. So, don't just make a living, make a life - don't just inhale, but breathe - don't just avoid death, but be alive. Be alive my friend, to all the unmanifested joy and cheer waiting to manifest through your actions - be alive to courage - be alive to conscience - be alive to liberation. Once you are alive to liberation, liberation would be alive in you. It's all simply a matter of realization, nothing more. It's a matter of realization beyond the labels that the society has imposed on you as a part of your identity. See those labels - try - try to see them as they are - try to see their innate sectarian and destructive nature. Can you? If you can, then all you need to do is to take that one big step into the land of true psychological liberation and oneness.

Liberation - it's a fine word, yet you can't even imagine what it's like to live in liberation with your second-hand existence as second-hand beings. You must first die to that existence with all its petty tribal traits, then and then only, will liberation reveal itself to you. With liberation comes strength, with liberation comes clarity, with liberation comes insight. And this insight is the real enlightenment with limitless potential to do good in the world, and in fact with the potential to make the words "good" and "world" intertwined. This insight has no mystical nonsense in it - it has no copyright of ownership belonging to a certain messiah or prophet. It's just plain human wisdom born from neurochemicals for the betterment of the human world.

Enlightenment is no mystical phenomenon, it's a purely psychological phenomenon born from the physical bases of neurons. Enlightenment that proclaims to be mystical in nature is nothing but the product of a mind swayed by ignorance, delusions and superstitions. Real enlightenment is not at all free from all sorts of ignorance, but it is at all times aware of that ignorance as well as all the shortcomings of the self, whereas in the so-called enlightenment fueled by mysticism, the self gets consumed by the illusion of knowledge, which is worse than ignorance.

Ignorance is healthy, as it keeps us moving ahead toward knowledge, but illusion of knowledge keeps us from growing - it turns us into a soul-less stone filled with barbarian stereotypes and prejudices. Here are some of the most disgusting illusions of knowledge that keep tormenting the society and impede in its progress even in this day and age.

- The world was created a few thousand years ago by a Super-Intelligent Being;
- All Muslims are terrorists;
- Global warming is a myth created by scientists;
- Vaccination is dangerous for the kids.

These are some of the most dangerous illusions of knowledge that unfortunately many of the so-called modern, smart and civilized humans believe to be factual truth. If you do not know the answer to a question, then first accept that you do not know and then try to find a rational answer, but never take beliefs as knowledge.

The difference between belief and knowledge is that, belief is personal, whereas knowledge is universal. A belief can become knowledge if it can be justified with rational thinking. If a belief is not backed up by reasoning then it has nothing to do with the society beyond the bounds of the individual mind holding the belief. An individual can foster as much absurd beliefs as the limbic heart desires, but if the person wants internal growth, then discarding the primitive irrational beliefs is imperative. Beliefs can be healthy as well as harmful. A modern mind must keep its faculty of reasoning active at all times in order to get rid of the harmful beliefs, so that they don't replace knowledge with illusion of knowledge.

Illusion no matter how sophisticated, can never take the place of knowledge, Yet the unfortunate reality of this world is, some people do indeed take their illusions, hallucinations and imaginations to be the real thing. This way, they not only delude themselves, but also their society, because humans are social animals, and as such they have an innate urge to share their personal beliefs, understandings and experiences that they deem important. Through this process, one person's delusion becomes the delusion of a people. And such delusions in time bring down catastrophe upon the world. So never accept a single word from your environment without properly filtering it with your rational mind.

However, as a doctor, you may often need to entertain the patient's belief, without actually accepting it to be factually true, if you see a potential positive impact of that belief in the person's recovery. So, as a doctor, you must be conscientious enough to distinguish a healthy belief from an unhealthy belief. For example, you may know that there is no supreme being that may restore health in a patient's body, but still, you must be ready to approve and even advocate for prayer if the patient desires to do so.

In a study of 40 patients who had heart transplants, strong religious beliefs predicted improved physical functioning, higher self-esteem, decreased anxiety, and enhanced compliance. Also, it has been shown that increased worship is inversely related to perception of disability among the elderly. In cancer patients, religious belief has been found to be associated with reduced perception of pain. Researchers have even found a relationship between religious activity and mortality. For example, multiple studies published in the 1980s and 1990s identified a correlation between frequent church attendance and a reduction in all-cause mortality.

In a study of 232 patients undergoing cardiac surgery, patients receiving support from religion had reduced mortality. Religiousness among cancer survivors is associated with positive health habits and social and emotional support. Cardiac patients identify religion and prayer as a frequently used coping mechanism prior to surgery.

Prayer and meditation can induce the relaxation response, which includes lower heart rate and blood pressure. This is mediated by activity in the anterior pituitary-adrenocortical axis. In fact, when a person engages in a blissful practice such as prayer or meditation, different regions of your brain light up like the night of Christmas Eve.

Increased activity in the limbic system, especially the thalamus counts for the intense divine ecstasy, which is an extremely heightened emotional mental state. And when one practices such rituals or prayer activity in communion, the event strengthens the entire heavenly experience for every single person in the communion. This also increases the neural connections of one's faith upon the divine to a great extent, which in turn impacts every single aspect of one's daily life.

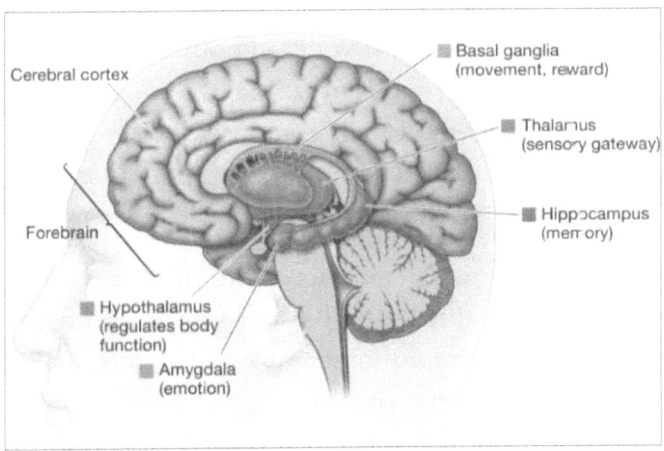

Figure 1.1 The Limbic System surrounded by the layers of Cerebral Cortex

The rhythms of one's prayer rituals impact over one's body physiologically. Your body is always overwhelmed with various biological rhythms. You have a heart rhythm, breathing rhythm, hormonal rhythms, and brain-wave rhythms. On top of that, when you experience an external rhythm such as a prayer or a religious song, your body's rhythms can actually begin to synchronize with the prayer or religious song.

Furthermore, as you engage in the rhythm, you start to feel it within your body. The rhythmic activity starts to drive your body and brain. Such activity drives your hypothalamus and, ultimately, your amygdala to generate inexplicable emotional responses. Fast music makes you feel excited and happy; slow music makes you feel calm and content.

And as all your emotions are tied to your thoughts, you incorporate the feelings into your cognition. Thus, the moment one has a thought about the importance of divine presence in one's life and connect it with a ritual that generates a strong feeling of happiness or love, one's brain begins to impregnate one's thoughts connected to the divine with positive emotions.

The moment a person embraces the amazing emotional sensation of rituals such as prayer or meditation, he or she embarks on an ever-positive journey toward better health. Prayer and meditation result in decreased heart rate, blood pressure, metabolism, and hormonal changes. Also, they result in increased serotonin, dopamine, and gamma-aminobutyric acid (GABA), which are the body's natural antianxiety drugs, and decreased cortisol and norepinephrine.

Many of the studies carried out by us neuroscientists show that long-term practice of meditation leads to emotional stability. Rituals such as prayer and meditation produce profound feelings of excitement or relaxation, depending on the nature of the ritual. If it is an intensely energetic and fast ritual, then they might induce great arousal. If it is an intensely calming and slow ritual, then they induce an overwhelming bliss. These experiences are mediated by the autonomic nervous system.

The physiology of a ritual is based on the rhythms synchronizing the brain in such a way that they begin to actually diminish the usual flow of sensory information entering the brain. And when you stimulate your brain in a very specific rhythm of the ritual, its normal sensory functioning begins to shift.

In this process, the mutual activation of the arousal and calming parts of the autonomic nervous system leads to the profound spiritual experience of ecstasy. Through the autonomic nervous system, the rhythm of your ritual causes some amazing alterations in your brain chemistry such as, increased activity in the hypothalamus, thalamus, and the whole limbic system. And this entire process of neurochemical activity, leads to a sustained internal wellbeing of the patient, which often leads to faster recovery.

Also, on the topic of prayers or any other personal ritual of the patient, you must appear to be least skeptical. Your behavior matters to the patient's psychological as well as physiological wellbeing, more than the behavior of any other person, for you are not an ordinary person, you are the caretaker of your patient's life, which is not merely a professional duty, but it is a divine responsibility, for divinity lies in sustaining lives, which is the very purpose of your life.

The best kind of existence is to exist for others. And it applies to you, the doctor, more accurately than any other person on earth. The very purpose of your life is to live for others. And if you don't still realize this simple revelation at the very core of your being, then my friend, I'm afraid that you are not yet ready to become a doctor. Doctorhood is not just yet another profession, it is the only profession that can literally breathe life into a dying soul. And that is no petty matter of money-making, it is a matter of utmost divinity, it is a matter of utmost practical godliness - the godliness that actually involves living, real gods, and not some imaginary gods.

You are a god, born to serve the gods in others, by treating their soul. Treating the body is only a portion of the entire process. And by soul, I'm not mentioning some supernatural force that uses the body as a vessel, rather I am talking about something much deeper than mystical stupidity. Born of neurons, soul is the very essence of being - soul is the very foundation of your existence - your psychological existence, from which all your physical prowess and progress manifest. Soul is the edifice of your being, which once born from the physical bases of protoplasm in the brain, can thereafter rewire and reorganize those very bases that it is born from, as it gains new experiences and insight.

Thus, the process of psychological evolution - the process of internal progress takes place in the deepest fathoms of the neuronal galaxy inside your skull. Neurons create soul, soul then reorganizes those neurons, then those reorganized neurons make the soul evolve. As such, it is nothing supernatural, but that does not make it any less awe-inspiring. In short, soul is a mish-mash, timey-wimey, weebly-wobley phenomenon of neurochemical magnificence. So, treat the soul my friend - treat the soul. Remember, a healthy body may or may not lead to a healthy soul, but a sick soul most certainly brings along sickness in the body.

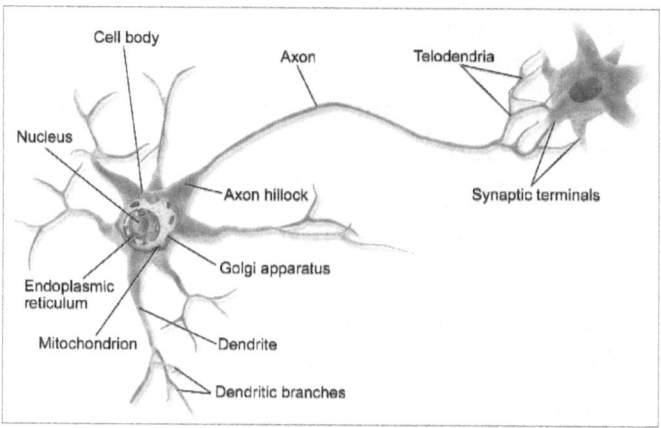

Figure 1.2 A Typical Neuron

Sickness is not merely a physiological phenomenon, hence, regardless of which kind of doctor you are, you must recognize sickness as it is, that is, a human phenomenon. Be aware of the whole domain of sickness - be aware of its implications in human life - be aware of its farthest reach in the life of the patient as well as the lives of the next of kin - be aware of its deepest roots, for that very awareness is the very foundation of true diagnosis, which automatically brings along the awareness of wellness.

Diagnosis is not a skill, it is an experience that slowly grows in you quite naturally, as you keep the gates of your soul open to the awareness of sickness. Understanding sickness in its whole form, reach and impact, automatically brings along the insight into wellness, just like understanding chaos with all its nuances brings along the true practical perception of harmony and the means to achieve it. And remember, wellness is not the lack of sickness, but the capacity to overcome sickness.

Sick are not those who possess a sickness, but those who are possessed by sickness. So, exorcise them with love, cheer and wisdom. Remember, there is no painkiller as effective as love, no anti-depressant as soothing as cheer, no defibrillator as powerful as wisdom. A doctor must have these fundamental elements flowing through his or her existence like cerebrospinal fluid.

A doctor should be a clown at heart, a scientist at brain and a mother at conscience. This means that a doctor should be cheerful, insightful and caring. Being cheerful does not mean always being funny, rather it means to be aware of the seriousness of a situation, and still keeping calm. Being insightful does not mean knowing everything about sickness and health, but to have the common mental maturity and capacity to accept when you do not know something, or to accept a mistake if committed. And being caring does not mean flattering or pampering the patient, but to genuinely take the wellbeing of the patient to be of more concern than the wellbeing of your own. And these three principal faculties of doctorhood grow stronger in time as you keep fostering and practising them. Practice of medicine is the collective practice of care, conscience and wisdom. And all that practice has one and one purpose only, it is to save, sustain and improve the value of life. A life saved is a family saved. And remember, human progress isn't measured by industry, it's measured by the value you put on a life.

What is life - life is not merely the functional expression of protoplasmic substance - it is the functional expression of protoplasmic substance that holds unimaginable potential for growth and progress. When you hold a bunch of seeds in your hand, all you can see with your physical eyes is a bunch of innocent seeds, but when you go beyond what your external eyes see, and try to grasp the true potential of those seeds, then and then only will you be able to see not just the seeds, but ginormous forests giving oxygen, shed and life to countless creatures on earth.

Sometimes to see the truth, you must turn blind to the obvious. And by blind I do not mean blindly believing in traditionally passed on beliefs and ideals, rather I mean to see beyond the perceptual capacities of those very traditions, ancient or modern – to see what those traditions can't see with their limited, either materialist or spiritualist perceptions. If you want to bring change, then you must not believe, rather you must perceive - perceive what others can't - imagine what others aren't capable of - and act in a way others wouldn't dare to.

You may advocate your patient's urge to pray for the benefit of the patient, but you must realize in your heart my friend, that there is no greater god in the entire world at that moment, capable enough to answer those prayers, than you. Remember, there never was any separate and supernatural trinity - it has always been the human mind playing the triangle, just like in dissociative identity disorder, but in a far more complicated and fantastic fashion. So, open your mind, recognize yourself and play God in the service of humanity.

It is either you a living creature of conscience plays God and saves lives, or some deluded monsters destroy lives on earth in the name of imaginary Gods and Angels. The choice is yours my friend. Arise upon the death of your second-hand existence - awake upon the permanent sleep of your conditioned life - and behave in the path of service - in the path of truth - in the path of liberty - behave, not like a worshiper, but as a God - the God - living God - the Mighty Human Being with infinite potential for greatness. Play God with all your might and conscience, because there is no greater Almighty than you the mighty and conscientious Human.

If you say, "let there be light", and then act with all your capacity to make it a reality, only then there will be light and hope in the world.

And this is no God complex - it would be, if you were to see yourself as superior to others, which you must not. You are not superior to anyone, except to those who see others as inferior. You are superior to those primordial imitations of human, the same way you are superior to a dog or a monkey. Advocating the supremacy of one's own groundless beliefs over others' is no sign of civilized and sentient human existence. If one is to exist as humans, one must first learn at one's very core of being, to act as humans.

And I believe, you can - act as novel, noble human. Remember, you are neither superior nor inferior to any other, for we all are human beings - with equal potential for greatness and glory. The only quality that distinguishes the greats from the rest of the population is their pride-less awareness of that greatness that lies in them. Once the humans implode with pride-less awareness, humanity will explode with egalitarian and progressive greatness.

You are full with seeds of greatness my friend. Just recognize them. Learn to see them beyond conflicting thoughts and opinions of both yourself and others. And once you do, you would become better at whatever you do. And this is no prophecy or assumption or speculation, rather it is an empirical reality of human psychological capacity. Perception creates possibility, and possibility creates reality. And the reality of human life is that your life is your decision - no imaginary monkey is going to come down on earth to say hello or give a hand in your times of need. So, you must be the hand that gives a hand to yourself when needed.

And when you are a doctor, you don't just need to give a hand to yourself, but your very hand becomes the prized possession of others. With your hands fortified with medical wisdom, you don't just treat, rather you heal. And the real medicine that heals the patient's soul is not the pharmaceuticals that you administer, rather it is your behavior – your interaction – your touch.

Your behavior holds the key to the effectiveness of your treatment. Treatment alone without the warm human side, is a nut without the kernel. Your warmth has more healing power upon the patient than all the medical tools in the world. Your warmth increases the effectiveness of your treatment, whereas your coldness would decrease that very effectiveness, for the body doesn't let any medicine work on it, unless the soul permits. And the permission of the patient's soul is granted only upon the encounter of your genuine warmth. That's the beauty of the effect of brain-body substrates which can be best explained by the process called the placebo effect.

The last decades have seen a significant increase in research endeavors that attempt to identify and understand processes relevant to the seemingly enigmatic phenomenon of placebo. By definition, placebo refers to a reduction in a symptom in an individual that results from one's perception of the therapeutic intervention. This response is the product of a fascinating twosome between biology and psychology. Placebo effect involves expectation, optimism and other states of motivational, emotional or cognitive appetence. These states appear to initiate partial beneficial effects through neural mechanisms that engage brain-body substrates to alter bodily processes.

Placebo effects rely on complex neurobiological mechanisms involving neurotransmitters (e.g., endorphins, cannabinoids and dopamine) and activation of specific relevant areas of the brain (e.g., prefrontal cortex, anterior insula, rostral anterior cingulate cortex and amygdala). Many common medications also act through these pathways. In addition, genetic signatures of patients who are likely to respond to placebos are beginning to be identified.

Such basic biological discoveries have greatly enhanced the credibility of placebo effects. Moreover, recent clinical research into placebo effects has provided compelling evidence that these effects are genuine neuropsychological phenomena.

Placebo interventions do not by definition, have any direct therapeutic effects on the body. However, all treatments are delivered in a context that includes social and physical cues, verbal suggestions and treatment history. This context is actively interpreted by the brain and can elicit expectations, memories and emotions, which in turn can influence health-related outcomes in the brain and body. Placebo effects are thus brain–body responses to context information that promote health and well-being.

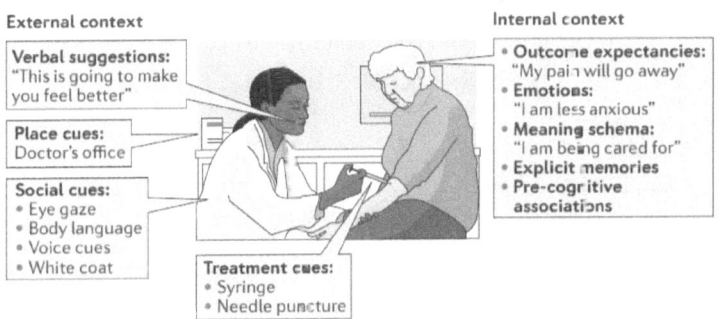

Figure 1.3 Elements of treatment context: Whether treatment consists of an active drug or a placebo, the clinical setting that surrounds treatment includes multiple types of context information that are perceived and interpreted by the patient's brain. The external context includes treatment, place and social cues, along with verbal suggestions. The internal context consists of memories, emotions, expectancies and appraisals of the meaning of the context for future survival and well-being. These features combine to make up the treatment context and are the 'active ingredients' of placebo effects. (Source: NATURE REVIEWS | Neuroscience Vol 16, July 2015)

And, when the brain's responses to context information, promote pain, distress and disease, instead of health, they are termed as "nocebo effects". Hence, the psychosocial factors that promote therapeutic placebo effects also have the potential to cause adverse consequences - nocebo effects.

Not infrequently, patients perceive side effects of medications that are actually caused by anticipation of negative effects or heightened attentiveness to normal background discomforts of daily life in the context of a new therapeutic regimen.

And as for placebos, though they may provide relief from certain heath issues by healing some of the symptoms, they rarely cure. Although research has revealed objective neurobiological pathways and correlates of placebo responses. The evidence to date suggests that the therapeutic benefits associated with placebo effects do not alter the pathophysiology of diseases beyond their symptomatic manifestations. They primarily address subjective and self-appraised symptoms. For example, there is no evidence that placebos can shrink tumors. However, experiments demonstrate that common symptoms of cancer and side effects of cancer treatment (e.g., fatigue, nausea, hot flashes, and pain) are genuinely responsive to placebo treatments.

Placebo effects are not just about the dummy medicine or pills. It is the whole context of the treatment that makes a deep impact over the patient's neurobiology. For example, a recent study of episodic migraine demonstrated that when patients took Rizatriptan (10 mg) that was labeled "placebo" (a treatment that theoretically had "pure pharmacologic effects"), the outcomes did not differ from those in patients given placebos deceptively labeled "Rizatriptan" (pure expectation effect). However, when Rizatriptan was correctly labeled "Rizatriptan," its analgesic effect increased by 50%. Similar results have been observed when other drugs, including morphine, fentanyl, and diazepam, have been administered openly and covertly.

Almost all the Alternative treatments you hear about, such as Homeopathy, Acupuncture, faith-healing etc. are nothing more than placebo. Those alternative treatments may elevate one's health temporarily by the force of neurochemical processes of belief, but sooner than later the person gets sick again. Remember, if a healing technique is demonstrated to have curative properties in properly controlled double-blind trials, it ceases to be alternative. It simply becomes medicine.

For example, the Australian National Health and Medical Research Council conducted what certainly is the most thorough and independent evaluation of Homeopathy in its 200 year long history. And now it is a proven fact that Homeopathy is nothing more than placebo.

After assessing more than 1,800 studies on homeopathy, Australia's National Health and Medical Research Council was only able to find 225 that were rigorous enough to analyze. And a systematic review of these studies revealed "no good quality evidence to support the claim that homeopathy is effective in treating health conditions." Hence, people who choose only homeopathy while rejecting or delaying medical treatment put their health at risk.

Homeopathy is basically a system for dosing up on a dilute solution of water. It was dreamed up in the late 18th century as a way of boosting the body's "vital spirit". One of the central principles handed down by its founder Samuel Hahnemann, was that "like cures like". Superficially this might sound vaguely plausible. But unlike a vaccine, that introduces a diminished form of a pathogen into the body in order to stimulate the immune system to develop adaptive immunity to that pathogen, "like cures like" makes the unfounded assumption, that what causes similar symptoms can cure those symptoms. In Hahnemann's magical world, dilute poison ivy cures skin rash because undiluted it causes a rash if touched. But amazingly homeopathy gets even stranger still.

Homeopaths claim that the more you dilute an active ingredient in water, the stronger medicine it becomes. Most homeopathic remedies are marked 30 C. It means 1 part medicine to 10030 parts of water. What would that mean in common words?

A drop in a fish-tank! No, a fish-tank is nowhere near big enough. Even a swimming pool doesn't provide enough dilution - not even a lake. What about a drop in the ocean! As it turns out, even the ocean isn't big enough.

For all the common homeopathic recipes, in order to get one molecule of the active substance, you need to drink all the atoms in the solar system. And to the rational mind, all of this, just doesn't make sense. Even Homeopaths acknowledge that there is not a single molecule of active ingredient in the bottle they sell you. It's just plain water. So, how can it possibly work!

In order to resolve the paradox, Homeopathy boldly paddles further up the creek of pseudoscience, claiming that the water somehow has a memory of the now completely absent active ingredient. In that case, wouldn't water also have memory of other more common impurities it's coming in contact with – salt, urine!

Scientists have calculated that in each glass of water we drink, at least one molecule has passed through the bladder of Letterman. Now you may ask, what about Ayurvedic remedies!

Ayurveda also falls under the category of Alternative medicine. But unlike the dilute solution of water, Ayurvedic remedies actually introduce active natural ingredients to the body. Ayurveda places more emphasis on prevention of illness and promotion of wellness, than on curing illness. And that's precisely what many of the Ayurvedic remedies do. Ingredients like ginger, honey, turmeric, cinnamon, clove, garlic etc. have in fact proven through countless studies to have significant influence in promoting health and preventing illness. However, even Ayurveda cannot be regarded as a substitute for modern medical treatment when it comes to treating a serious health issue.

Science has given us modern medicine. Now it is up to us, whether we embrace them like civilized, rational human beings, or cling to the ignorance, delusions and magical thinking of our ancestors. It is the modern medicine that treats diseases, not some alternative method of ancient treatment. Almost all the alternative treatments work through the power of the mind, and they only alleviate the symptoms temporarily. It is all in the brain.

The human brain is the most complex organized structure in the universe. It is the biological organ with mind-boggling capabilities, that you cannot even imagine. And the construction of beliefs is one of those capabilities. Your brain has the extraordinary ability to carry out fascinating neurochemical processes that can for a certain period of time transform your psychological belief into your physiological reality. And these processes result in either placebo effects or nocebo effects.

In short, taking a Homeopathic medicine, or visiting a faith-healing session, with the belief that it would relieve you from your certain health issue, can actually ease the symptoms for some time – but only for some time.

Now let me give you an example of nocebo effect. Say you visit a Doctor with an everyday illness. And he misdiagnoses your condition, by mixing up your reports with those of a Cancer patient, and tells you that you have Cancer. He also tells you that you only have a few months to live. In such scenario, after hearing this diagnosis, your brain would literally start anticipating the impending doom. And this anticipation would actually make you severely ill with every passing day, despite the fact that you never had Cancer. So, ultimately it is all about your belief. Through the brain-body substrates, your belief alone can either boost your immune system, or diminish it.

So, in short, if the patient believes in you, then the effectiveness of the treatment increases, but if the patient can't trust you, then no matter how good treatment you provide, its effectiveness will not be enough for the patient's recovery. So, the recovery of the patient is predicated on not just the treatment you provide, rather it is predicated literally on you. You are the patient's gateway to recovery, not the treatment. The treatment is only an essential portion of the equation of medical practice, but it is not the whole equation. Practice of medicine is not the practice of postponing death, rather it is the practice of improving the quality of life.

And this practice is rarely going to be easy - so, get rid of any such thoughts from your head in the first place, if you really want to be a doctor. Practice of medicine can take place only on the firm psychological ground of patience. Patience is the golden virtue in doctorhood. A patient doctor is a real doctor - an impatient doctor is no doctor at all.

And this patience must rise from your soul in a natural manner, not by force. But the fact of the matter is, when you begin your journey of medicine as a med student, it's very likely for you to not have that patience. So, you shall be required to foster the patience, that's already vested in your neurons, but lies unmanifested as the synaptic bonds required to make that patience rise to act, are not made yet. So, recognize the patience within you and then make it manifest with your genuine desire for doing good to your patients. Be persistent with your patience and it will grow stronger. And that very patience will make you a real doctor - a good doctor. A good doctor is a good person - every other kind of doctor is no doctor at all. And if you wonder what makes you a good doctor, then you are a good doctor.

In actuality, as a doctor, you don't practice medicine, rather you become the medicine yourself. You my friend, are the indomitable medicine at work, in the great service of humanity. You are humanity's first and last line of defense against all illness - but as I said earlier - your purpose is not to postpone death or delay the illness - your purpose is to improve the quality of life – and if you succeed in doing, even a little bit of it, then your practice of medicine is indeed a true success.

No one can defeat death, not even you - that's a fact of 21st century. Perhaps this fact would change in the coming millennia, as we solve the puzzle of neurodegeneration and find a way to merge the nervous system with a mechanical body, but for now, that is only a dream in the labs of a few scientists. So, for now my friend, all life is at your hands - your hands hold the priceless elixir of existence - your hands are the real hands of a messiah.

You are a messiah - recognize that, not in narcissistic self-absorbed manner, rather in a self-aware manner. Be aware of who you are and why you are here. There is a difference between how you live your life and what you do with it. So, choose, right now, what exactly is the purpose of your life, because without a clear insight into the unique purpose of your own unique life, there is no predestined purpose of life whatsoever, be it a human life or a non-human life, except for the purpose of survival.

So, don't just survive - live. Live for others as much as you live for yourself, for that is real living of a real sentient human. Human you are and your purpose is to radiate humanity. Humanity is bursting in you already - all you need to do is simply let it flood your actions. Think with humanity - feel with humanity - act with humanity.

Act, act and act again, for in your action lies emancipation for your kind. Your kind is not a civilized species - not yet - but it can be - it can be civilized - it can be conscientious - you just need to show it how. Your civilized actions will become the civilized actions of your kind - your conscientious footsteps will become the conscientious footsteps of your kind. Your glorious existence will become the reason for your kind to want to become better - to become civilized - to become conscientious.

You can't teach people to act conscientious - you can only become the living embodiment of conscience yourself, from which others would learn by themselves through the process of psychological osmosis. Be the ocean of conscience in which others can bathe. Be the sacred river of service, that takes away selfishness from the society. Be the mountain of bravery that absorbs weakness from the heart of people. And you must do all this as a humble servant as well as a pride-less leader of the people. Remember, pride is poison. It can ruin the greatness of the greatest of characters.

Pride is a form of euphoria in effect, that blinds the self to the shortcomings of the source of pride, by the inactivation of prefrontal cortex related to the matters of that source. It is a cognitive blindness that the blind is not even aware of. So, be aware before you turn blind - awareness keeps the blindness away. Be the paragon of awareness and all things great shall follow, both for you and your kind. Don't just be a doctor, be a doctor with awareness - don't just be a scientist, be a scientist with awareness - don't just be a preacher, be a preacher with awareness - don't just be a janitor, be a janitor with awareness - whatever you do, you must do it with awareness, or else, the force of life would run outta window.

When a doctor is blinded by pride, it doesn't only affect his or her own progress as a doctor, but more importantly it affects his or her capacity to treat the patient. When you are blinded by your pride of being a so-called extraordinary doctor, you may actually be committing real malpractice, by maltreating the patient, without ever being aware of it. So, always keep your compass of conscience on, so that, the moment pride begins to get hold of you, you get hold of your pride right back, before it can actually make you do any harm to the patient. Pride is blind, so it poisons your soul as a doctor, as well as a free human being.

Ask yourself - what is a free human being - what is a free human life - what is a free human consciousness! Don't expect me to tell you - just ask yourself - and be in the flow of asking - be the question and the answer will reveal itself. Answers are simple, it's just the humans who don't know how to ask the right question the right way. You may wonder, what is this so-called right way, if there is any such thing! Of course, you deserve to wonder - our ancestors went through the struggle for survival against the Monster Nature, so that we could wonder. And that's precisely it - to wonder - to wonder is to learn - to wonder is to grow - to wonder is to live. Live with wonder - because in the simplicity of wonder lie the answers.

And in order to wonder without judgement, you must expand your consciousness beyond the size of your society. Act with wonder, humility and regard for human frailty. You will never be a first-class doctor unless you learn to have some regard of human frailty, as I said earlier - and this regard appears naturally in you, if you have humility within. And humility comes through awareness of the depths of yourself. The ocean of self-awareness is teeming with jewels of wisdom and insight, but to discover them one must first accept death of one's identity. It is only when you become nothing, that you become alive and sentient.

Sentience creates bridge between people. Be sentient, not just in terms of biology, but in terms of actual psychological reality. Here I am not saying that biology is separate from psychology, rather I am saying that regardless of how much wonderful capacities you hold in your biology, unless you make them manifest in your actual everyday psychological reality, they are essentially useless. If you are not truly sentient in your psyche, no matter how many books of biological sciences proclaim that humans are sentient creatures, it won't matter the slightest bit in the actual sentient and humane progress of humanity. And a doctor is the one who ensures that this progress is a healthy one. And this is no petty professional duty, rather it is the supreme duty of a novel human soul.

Professionalism is a pompous myth, which only squeezes the life out of action. If an action doesn't have life in it, it has gone in waste. Don't waste your time and valuable potential on worthless tribalistic professionalism, rather bring all the powers of your nerves out and utilize them in the endeavor of excellence. Be not professional in what you do, rather be excellent. Excellence has life in it - it has colors in it - it has sweetness in it - whereas professionalism is a dead corpse exuding the disgusting smell of obedience. Excellence requires no obedience, yet in excellence you act your best, without all the life-sucking efforts. Now here arises the question - what is the nature of excellence!

The nature of excellence is effortlessness - the nature of excellence is action without anticipation for reward - the nature of excellence is living the flow of action. Excellence lies in everything that's not bound to desperation, prejudice and obedience. Excellence lies in freedom - excellence lies in all endeavors of the liberated mind. If you are free - if you have liberty in your soul - then excellence will kiss your feet without you making effort to achieve it. Excellence is not a fixed point in the future - excellence is a cease-less journey of evolution in the neurons. When neurons connect with each other, your mind excels in some aspect or other -

and when existing connections between neurons fade away, their correlated aspect of your psychological and behavioral existence fades away as well. So, it all depends on action - the more you act, the more you excel, for better or for worse. Excellence is predicated upon prideless, effortless and ambitionless action, not upon desperation, hopes and prayers. So, arise and act, and in time, excellence will manifest through you.

Now, I just said that excellence is predicated upon ambitionless action. Here one may wonder what's wrong with ambition! So, let's go deep into the matter. There is nothing wrong with ambition, but there is nothing glorious about it either. Ambition puts your mind in a state of high and keeps you running after an illusory goal, without actually letting you experience the flow of life. It's like the horse in the race that is kept running with blinders around its eyes only to win the race. You are not a race-horse, you are a human being - so, realize your true knacks and tastes and live them with all your grace. Don't let the childish clouds of ambition take away the life out of your existence.

It's not enough to exist - animals exist, but it's the humans who have the brain capacity to live. So, live my friend, without effort, without worry, without ambition, without pride - live with dignity, contentment and the idea that gives your life value. If you truly genuinely want to do something, you just do it - just like the river flows without having any ambition to flow - the sun doesn't have an ambition to shine - it is in the ambition-less, pride-less, non-judgmental, non-conceptual, non-conflicting flow of action, that lies the force of life. So, flow like the river - shine like the sun - if you want to live - then live without the run.

Remember, it is better to die while living, than to live while dying. There is life in walking, but death in running - there is life in communication, but death in talking - there is life in awareness, but death in judgement - so, be the life my friend, without the judgement, without the talking, without the running - simply be the life, full with sparkling communications, revelatory awareness and heart-warming walks. Take it slow and be the flow. Flow all day, every day, without the rush to get anywhere - simply flow - and in that flow you shall truly begin to see yourself, like you've never seen before - in that flow your soul will become the breeding ground of all excellence - of all greatness - of all glory. Glory, excellence and greatness all come when you stop seeking them. Stop seeking and start acting, because the seeker only gets lost in the process of seeking, never to realize the fact that once you cease the urge to seek, what you seek appears to you by itself.

The process of seeking leads to an amputated spirit. Prosthetics can fix physical disabilities. But no prosthetic can fix an amputated spirit. So, don't let the society strip you of your own spirit. Be brave and upright, and delve even into the depth of doom to achieve your goal, and you must do it with grace, simplicity and awareness. If you need to force yourself to do something, you shouldn't do it in the first place. Do it with your spirit, or not at all. Only then we shall see the rise of a world full of free humans.

The very nature of these free humans is compassion, kindness and acceptance - these free humans wouldn't even feel the slightest instinctual inclination to discriminate others on the basis of race, religion and nationality. To these humans all are humans, and nothing less than humans. To these humans a black person, is not a black person, but a human - to these humans a brown person, is not a brown person, but a human - to these humans, a white person, is not a white person, but a human - to these humans a christian, or a jew, or a muslim, or an atheist, is not a christian, jew, muslim or atheist, rather they all simply are humans - and this could only happen with the rise of true, genuine, psychological oneness - oneness that makes you see yourself in others. If you can't see yourself in others, then psychologically, there is not much difference between you and the animals.

Bring your entire psychological force into action and contemplate upon the question - what makes us humans! We breathe air in from our environment - we consume nutrition from mother nature, in the form of food and water - we copulate and reproduce to keep our genetic heritage alive through time - but is this enough to make us humans! Because, if breathing, eating, copulating and reproducing - these acts made us humans, then the dogs on the streets would be as much humans as we are - but surely we are not like the dogs - we are different from the dogs - and indeed from any other animal on earth. So, what does distinguish us, from other animals!

Technically we are animals, in terms of biological sciences - but we are not going into these technicalities - we are trying to go deep into the understanding of what makes us humans. Think - why are we different from the animals! We are different from the animals because, unlike the animals we can recognize our errors - the animals do have traces of this trait but only enough to avoid danger and ensure survival - but we on the other hand, are way more advanced in this capacity of recognizing our shortcomings, much beyond survival needs.

We can recognize our mistakes, and then think over them and act accordingly in order to eliminate them from our characteristics and become better. Now what would you call this very process of recognizing our shortcomings and mistakes and becoming better! Isn't this the thing we called "awareness" - "self-awareness". There is nothing mystical in all this - there's no mystical mumbo-jumbo involved here - just plain ordinary awareness - awareness of ourselves - of our thoughts - of our emotions - of our behavior. And the more we are aware of ourselves, the more we get to be truly humans - because without that awareness, we are just the same as the animals.

That very awareness makes you think that when you are kind to others, it would create a humane world - perhaps not for yourselves, but for your children and their children. So, with awareness we begin - we take that first step towards eliminating the distance between two people - you and the other, beyond all labels of profession, religion, race, nationality and everything else. So, in the truest sense of the term, when awareness rises from the human mind, the distance among the humans vanishes, thus rises oneness - in that oneness lies true compassion - in that oneness lies true union of all humanity.

That union doesn't even need the word "compassion" to explain itself, because you would by your very nature, be kind to the other person, as you would not see that other person as a different person, but simply an image of yourself. All humans are images of your own self - once you recognize this simple fact, there would no longer be any hatred - there would no longer be any prejudice in the world - there will simply be compassion - there will simply be kindness. When that oneness rises - compassion will not need human efforts to be spread, because oneness is compassion - compassion is kindness - kindness is empathy - empathy is morality - morality is spirituality - and spirituality is religion - all these terms are created by humans without them even being aware of the fact that it all comes down to one simple sense of oneness.

With that oneness burning bright in your core of being, you get to be the human replete with compassion, courage and conscience. And when these three real trinity flow pure and strong in your veins, you become a real healer to the society, and then, whatever you do, brings serenity in the world - it brings warmth in the world - it brings health, prosperity and progress in the world.

Right action radiates from you when oneness manifests in your mind. And with that right action, you will create with your own hands, the right course of human history. History doesn't exist, except in the memory of humans, and as such it can't be changed. The course of history however, is a different story, for it is the path that humanity is walking on right now, and as such it is in the hands of the humans to shape it the way they want.

Think over it - what is history! Think – slowly. History exists only in the memory of us humans – it exists in our neurons. So, outside of us, history doesn't exist, other than the remnants of it, such as all those heritage sites, statues and others. Now, can one person change history. We just said that history doesn't exist, so, if it doesn't exist, there is no question of changing it – but a human being does have the capacity, unlike any other animal, to actually change the course of history, which means change the path, or rather make the path, on which we are going. Therefore, we do have the capacity to create history right now, which will be seen as history by the people of the future. So, we can't change history, but we can change the course of evolution.

Now think about this, for the first time, in the history of life on earth, one species has gained the brain capacity to actually consciously choose the path of its own evolution, influence its own evolution- that's us – Homo sapiens – more than seven billion of them. Now, imagine. what if you truly become aware of your capacities – you become aware of what you can really do – you become aware of the potential that lies unmanifested within your nerves! You would literally start creating history at this very moment – because you would be creating the future.

The only way to change the course of history is to create the future right now, so that the people of tomorrow will look back at you and at the very least, they will not be ashamed of you, all because you stepped beyond instinctual primitiveness and acted with conscientious footsteps. They will even be proud of you – you the humanity of today – for your actions, the right kind of actions – the actions that bring true, genuine, humane progress among all humans. Freedom doesn't mean doing whatever you want - freedom means doing what brings warm, humane progress for the self as well as others. So, the right impact of freedom is predicated upon right action.

In action lies life, and with that action, history is made. It is as simple as that. Empirically speaking, there is no such thing as history, destiny and even future for that matter, what there really is, is the "now". And this very "now" – this very moment is the only thing which you have in your hands – in fact, it is the only time that actually exists – the "now". So, be aware of that "now" and you will literally begin to see all moments like a true seer, without all the mystical nonsense. Simply awareness will make you see, what has been, what will be and what could be.

Then comes the choice – the choice of action, but again when I say choice of action – it would manifest as a natural step to take to the free soul, which means there would be no alternative. Because the real choice is in choicelessness, so the alternative doesn't even appear to you – what appears to you when you are truly aware and free is the right action – and that right action manifests through you – because outside you actions don't exist, outside you history doesn't exist, outside you future doesn't exist. So, all the world, all events, all phenomena in the human universe, rise from you, within you, in your neurons. And the most vibrant way to understand this neurological revelation, is through the observation of various mind-boggling neurological syndromes.

Brain circuits with various neurological conditions (fatal or harmless) can completely alter one's conscious perception of the reality. The perception of reality is often referred to as "Qualia" in the neuroscientific community. Qualia (plural form of "quale") are the raw feelings of conscious experience such as, the taste of your lover's lips, smell of his/her body, the redness of red, the painfulness of pain etc. Synesthesia is such an extraordinary neurological phenomenon, where an individual's physical senses get mixed up. Sensations evoked through one sensory pathway produce vivid qualia normally associated with another physical sense. Perhaps it would be easier for you to understand if I mention the experiences of synesthesia. Individuals with this condition report physically 'seeing' sounds/smells/tastes or 'tasting' colors/sounds or 'hearing' colors and so on.

However some forms of synesthesia can occur during stages of meditation, sensory deprivation or even during the use of psychedelics such as LSD, marijuana etc. And the biological cause behind synesthesia is merely cross-connection between different brain regions of the somatosensory system involved in different sensory functions.

Conscious awareness of the reality is a mysterious thing. Cognitive reality of an individual solely arises from the make-up of that individual's brain structure. Any kind of damage, like stroke can alter this reality without the awareness of the individual. Let me tell you a story of a stroke patient with such an altered cognitive reality. Her condition was noticed by my friend and colleague V.S. Ramachandran, one of the most interesting neuroscientists of our times. He explains her condition like this:

> *"Who was this rolling out of the bedroom in a wheelchair? Sam couldn't believe his eyes. His mother, Ellen, had just returned home the night before, having spent two weeks at the Kaiser Permanente hospital recuperating from a stroke. Mom had always been fastidious about her looks. Clothes and makeup were Martha Stewart perfect, with beautifully coiffed hair and fingernails painted in tasteful shades of pink or red. But today something was seriously wrong. The naturally curly hair on the left side of*

Ellen's head was uncombed, so that it stuck out in little nestlike clumps, whereas the rest of her hair was neatly styled. Her green shawl was hanging entirely over her right shoulder and dragging on the floor. She had applied rather bright red lipstick to her upper right and lower right lips, leaving the rest of her mouth bare. Likewise, there was a trace of eyeliner and mascara on her right eye but the left eye was unadorned. The final touch was a spot of rouge on her right cheek—

very carefully applied so as not to appear as if she were trying to hide her ill health but enough to demonstrate that she still cared about her looks. It was almost as though someone had used a wet towel to erase all the makeup on the left side of his mother's face!

"Good grief!" cried Sam. "What did you do to your makeup?"

Ellen raised her eyebrow in surprise. What was her son talking about? She had spent half an hour getting ready this morning and felt she looked as good as she possibly could, given the circumstances.

Ten minutes later, as they sat eating breakfast, Ellen ignored all the food on the left side of her plate, including the fresh-squeezed orange juice she so loved.

Sam raced for the phone and called me (Ramachandran), as one of the physicians who had spent time with his mother at the hospital. Sam and I had gotten to know one another while I had been seeing a stroke patient who shared a room with his mother. "It's all right," I said, "don't be alarmed. Your mother is suffering from a common neurological syndrome called hemi-neglect, a condition that often follows strokes in the right brain, especially in the right parietal lobe. Neglect patients are profoundly indifferent to objects and events in the left side of the world, sometimes including the left side of their own bodies."

"You mean she's blind on the left side?"

"No, not blind. She just doesn't pay attention to what's on her left. That's why we call it neglect."

The next day I was able to demonstrate this to Sam's satisfaction by doing a simple clinical test on Ellen. I sat directly in front of her and said,

"Fixate steadily on my nose and try not to move your eyes." When her gaze was fixed, I held my index finger up near her face, just to the left of her nose, and wiggled it vigorously.

"Ellen, what do you see?"

"I see a finger wiggling," she replied.

"Okay," I said. "Keep your eyes fixed on the same spot on my nose." Then, very slowly and casually, I raised the same finger to the same position, just left of her nose. But this time I was careful not to move it abruptly. "Now what do you see?"

Ellen looked blank. Without having her attention drawn to the finger—via motion or other strong cues—she was oblivious. Sam began to understand the nature of his mother's problem, the important distinction between blindness and neglect. His mother would ignore him completely if he stood on her left side and did nothing. But if he jumped up and down and waved his arms, she would sometimes turn around and look.

For the same reason, Ellen fails to notice the left side of her face in a mirror, forgets to apply makeup on the left side of her face, and doesn't comb her hair or brush her teeth on that side. And, not surprisingly, she even ignores all the food on the left side of her plate. But when her son points to things in the neglected area, forcing her to pay attention, Ellen might say, "Ah, how nice. Fresh-squeezed orange juice!" or "How embarrassing. My lipstick is crooked and my hair unkempt."

...

Finally, I took a sheet of paper, put it in front of Ellen and asked her to draw a flower.

"What kind of flower?" she said.

"Any kind. Just an ordinary flower."

Again, Ellen paused, as if the task were difficult, and finally drew another circle. So far so good. Then she painstakingly drew a series of little petals—it was a daisy—all scrunched on the right side of the flower (Figure 1.4)."

Such neglect is not blindness, rather it is simply a general indifference to objects and events on the left. Let me give you another similar yet a little different kind of neglect case history.

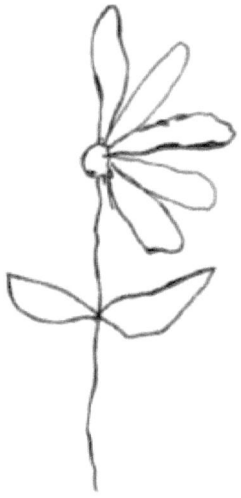

Figure 1.4 Drawing made by the hemineglect patient. Notice that the left half of the flower is missing. Many neglect patients will also draw only half the flower when drawing from memory— even with their eyes closed. This implies that the patient has also lost the ability to "scan" the left side of the internal mental picture of the flower. (Ramachandran, 1996)

A schoolteacher suffered a stroke that paralyzed the left side of her body, but she insists that her left arm is not paralyzed. Once, when she was asked, whose arm was lying in the bed next to her, she explained that the limb belonged to her brother. Then, when she was asked to clap, she proceeded to make clapping movements with her right hand, as if clapping with an imaginary left hand near the midline, while her left hand kept lying completely paralyzed with no movement whatsoever.

This patient was in fact completely paralyzed on the left side of her body after a stroke that damaged the right hemisphere of her brain. And like this one there is a small subset of patients with right hemispheric damage who seem to be absolutely unaware of the fact that the entire left side of their body is paralyzed even though they are quite mentally lucid in all other aspects. In the year 1908 French neurologist Joseph François Babinski first observed this curious disorder in which the patient's tendency is to ignore or sometimes even to deny the fact that one's left arm or leg is paralyzed. Babinski termed this condition as "Anosognosia" that means "unaware of illness".

Neglect stories are very popular in the field of neurology. There is another kind of neglect or denial in which a person downright denies to be alive. Yes, you heard right! It is another fascinating neurophychiatric syndrome called "Cotard" or "walking corpse" syndrome.

This syndrome was named after the French neurologist Jules Cotard. He described the condition as 'le délire de negation' or 'the delirium of negation'. It results in a feeling that one is either dead or immortal. In 1880 Jules Cotard reported the case of a 43 year old lady, Mademoiselle X who believed that she had "no brain, nerves, chest or entrails and was just skin and bone", that "neither God nor the devil existed" and that "she was eternal and would live forever". The syndrome is described to have various degrees of severity, ranging from mild to severe. In a mild state, feelings of despair and self-loathing occur, whereas in the severe state the person with Cotard syndrome actually starts to deny the very existence of the self. In 2007 McKay and Cipolotti published a report on a 24 year old patient called LU. LU repeatedly thought that she was in heaven, even though she was actually in National Hospital, Queen Square, London and that she might have died from flu. The delusions diminished over a few days and were gone after a week.

Cotard delusion is usually associated with lesions in the parietal lobe as well as the prefrontal cortex. It can be treated with various antipsychotic, antidepressant and mood stabilizing drugs along with electroconvulsive therapy (ECT) and psychotherapy. The brain of an individual with Cotard syndrome, generates the conscious awareness of being dead. However, such delusion does not hamper one's daily choirs and the person walks around and carries out daily activities just like a normal healthy person. The delusion goes away with treatment, but until it vanishes, it remains the only conscious reality to the person.

However, I must make something clear here. Individuals with these mental illnesses cannot be considered as "crazy", since they are completely lucid in all other daily activities. These mental conditions are simply emergency defense measures constructed by the subconscious to deal with sudden overwhelming bewilderments about one's body and the space around it.

There is another mind-boggling neurological phenomenon, called Capgras' syndrome, where the patient sees familiar and loved figures as impostors. This delusion is one of the rarest and most colorful syndromes in neurology. The patient, who is often mentally quite lucid, comes to regard close acquaintances, usually his parents, children, spouse or siblings, as impostors. One patient reported with absolute belief: *"That man looks identical to my father but he really isn't my father. That woman who claims to be my mother? She's lying. She looks just like my mom but it isn't her."* Many of the documented cases of Capgras' syndrome have occurred in association with traumatic brain injury. This implies that the syndrome has a neurological basis.

Capgras' delusion results from a disconnection between the face recognition region in the temporal lobe and the emotion center of the brain, i.e. amygdala. Face recognition pathways remain completely normal, so a person with Capgras' could identify everyone, but as the communication between the face recognition region and amygdala is selectively damaged he/she would not experience any emotions when looking at the faces of his/her beloved ones. In the case of the patient mentioned earlier, he doesn't feel a "warm glow" when looking at his beloved mother, so when he sees her he says to himself, *"If this is my mother, why doesn't her presence make me feel like I'm with my mother?"* So the only way he could make sense of it, is to subconsciously assume that this woman merely resembles his Mom, but is actually an impostor, which then becomes a part of his conscious cognitive reality.

Often the brain of a person with Capgras' delusion creates some really bizarre cognitive reality. In one of such recorded case histories, a patient was convinced that his stepfather was a robot, proceeded to decapitate him and opened his skull to look for microchips.

But why exactly the close relatives are perceived as imposters and not any other familiar face? This is because when a person encounters someone who is emotionally very close to him/her, such as a parent, spouse or sibling, he/she naturally expects an emotional glow, a warm fuzzy feeling. The absence of this glow in the most expected relationship is therefore surprising which is then rationalized by the subconscious part of the mind through an absurd delusion. On the other hand, when a person sees someone familiar but not emotionally close, he/she doesn't expect a warm glow and consequently there is no need for the brain to generate a delusion to explain the lack of warm and fuzzy feeling.

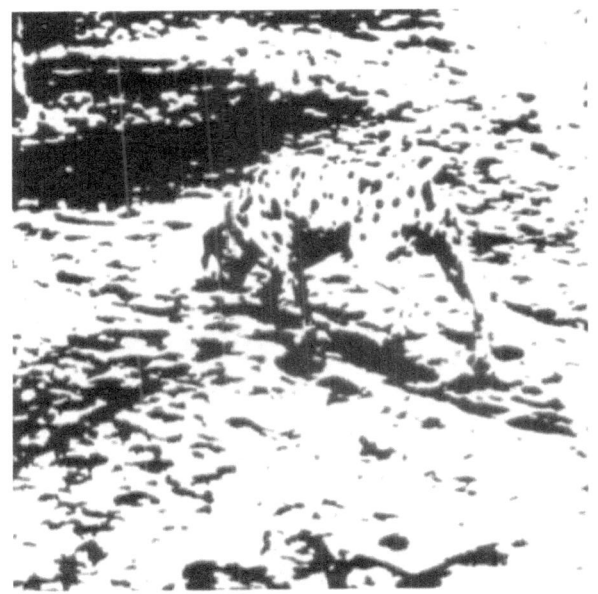

Figure 1.5 Random jumble of splotches. Gaze at this picture for a few seconds and you will eventually see a Dalmatian dog sniffing the ground mottled with shadows of leaves. Once the dog has been seen, it is impossible to get rid of it. Neurons in the temporal lobes become altered permanently after the initial brief exposure, once you have "seen" the dog. (Tovee, Rolls and Ramachandran, 1996)

Observing the medical histories of various neurological syndromes is like observing human nature and human consciousness through a magnifying lens. They remind us of the overwhelming aspects of human silliness. They make us realize how easily our own mind can play tricks on us.

The human construct of the so-called reality is prone to self-deception. One way or another, we all are being deceived by our own mind. We always see what we want to see. Every moment, we create a new reality, and then the earlier reality loses its accountability (Figure 1.5).

Perception of reality emerges from the brain and dissolves in the brain. All your hopes, happiness, aspirations and inspirations rise from the intricate and enchanting neural firings in your brain. Those neurons can create time – they can destroy time – those neurons can create future, they can destroy future – those neurons can create a beautiful world, they can also create a horrible planet to live on – those neurons are both the pedestrians and the path of truth and liberty. And as you keep walking on that path, you walk as your neurons – and every single step that you take could either be the beacon of hope and health, above all conscience to all humanity, or it could be a gruesome scar in the memory of humanity. So, don't just walk my friend, walk wisely. The world has enough smartness, in the form of doctors and many other professions, but what the world really needs is love, warmth and wisdom, through whichever profession you see fit.

Hence, you should not become a doctor, because you love medicine, you should become a doctor, because you love humanity. Without the love for humanity, no doctor is a doctor, but only a valueless imitation of a doctor. A doctor's value should not be measured simply by his or her understanding of medicine, rather it should be measured by his or her concern for the wellbeing of humanity.

And mark this my friend, there may be medical tools in your hands to treat the patient, but those hands must be that of a loving, warm and conscientious human being. The world doesn't need more smart doctors, it needs more warm and wise doctors. Be the wisdom yourself - be the warmth yourself, and be the doctor that the doctors have forgotten to be, for it is time to save medicine, to save humanity.

BIBLIOGRAPHY

Aristotle. Politics. Penguin; Revised, Reprint edition. (2000)

Aristotle. De Anima (On the Soul). Penguin Random House. 1987

Aristotle. Physics. Kessinger Publishing, 2004

Adolphs R (2003) Cognitive neuroscience of human social behaviour. Nature Rev Neurosci 4: 165–178.

Adolphs R, Tranel D, Damasio AR (2003) Dissociable neural systems for recognizing emotions. Brain Cogn 52: 61–69.

Allison T, Puce A, McCarthy G. (2000) Social perception from visual cues: role of the STS region. Trends Cogn Sci 4: 267–278.

Ashbrook, James, and Carol Albright. The Humanizing Brain: Where

Religion and Neuroscience Meet. Cleveland, OH: Pilgrim Press, 1997.

Azari, Nina, Janpeter Nickel, Gilbert Wunderlich, Michael Niedeggen, Harald Hefter, Lutz Tellmann, Hans Herzog, Petra Stoerig, Dieter Birnbacher, and Rudiger Seitz. "Neural Correlates of Religious Experience." European Journal of Neuroscience 13, no. 8 (2001)

Agar, N. (2004). Liberal eugenics: In defence of human enhancement. London: Blackwell Publishing.

Alteheld, N., Roessler, G., Vobig, M., & Walter, R. (2004). The retina implant new approach to a visual prosthesis. Biomedizinische Technik, 49(4), 99–103.

Antal, A., Nitsche, M. A., Kincses, T. Z., Kruse, W., Hoffmann, K. P., & Paulus, W. (2004a). Facilitation of visuo-motor learning by transcranial direct current stimulation of the motor and extrastriate visual areas in humans. European Journal of Neuroscience, 19(10), 2888–2892.

Augustine JR (1996) Circuitry and functional aspects of the insular lobe in primates including humans. Brain Res Rev 22: 229–244.

Bacon, F. (1803). The works of Francis bacon, baron of Verulam, viscount

St Alban, and lord high chancellor of England. London: H. Bryer.

Bacon, F. (1874). The advancement of learning. In J. Spedding, R. L.

Ellis, & D. D. Heath (Eds.), The philosophical works of Francis Bacon

(Vol. III). London: Longman.

Beauchamp, T. L., & Childress, J. F. (2009). Principles of biomedical ethics (6th ed.). New York: Oxford University Press.

Beauchamp, T. L. (2008). The principle of beneficence in applied ethics.

Barash, D. P. (1977). Sociobiology of rape in mallards (Anas platyrhynchos): Responses of the mated male. - Science 197, p. 788-789.

Barthalomew, G. A. (1970). A model for the evolution of pinniped polygyny. - Evolution 24, p. 546-559.

Berger, J. (1986). Wild horses of the great basin: Social competition and population size. - The University of Chicago Press, Chicago.

Birkhead, T. R., Johnson, S. D. & Nettleship, D. N. (1985). Extra-pair matings and mate guarding in the common murre Uria aalge. - Anim. Behav. 33, p. 608-619.

Beauregard, Mario, and Vincent Paquette. "Neural Correlates of a Mystical Experience in Carmelite Nuns." Neuroscience Letters 405, no. 3 (2006)

Benson, Herbert. Timeless Healing: The Power and Biology of Belief. New York: Scribner, 1996

Bogen, J.E.(1995a), 'On the neurophysiology of consciousness: Part I. An overview', Consciousness and Cognition, 4.

Bogen, J.E. (1995b), 'On the neurophysiology of consciousness: Part II. Constraining the semantic problem', Consciousness and Cognition, 4.

Bremner, J. D., R. Soufer, et al. (2001). "Gender differences in cognitive and neural correlates of remembrance of emotional words." Psychopharmacol Bull 35 (3).

Brothers, L. (2002). The social brain: A project for integrating primate behavior and neurophysiology in a new domain. In J. T. Cacioppo et al. (Eds.), Foundations in neuroscience. Cambridge, MA: MIT Press.

Buss, D. D. (2003). Evolutionary Psychology: The New Science of Mind, 2nd ed. New York: Allyn & Bacon.

Buss, D. M. (1989). "Conflict between the sexes: Strategic interference and the evocation of anger and upset." J Pers Soc Psychol 56 (5).

Buss, D. M. (1995). "Psychological sex differences. Origins through sexual selection." Am Psychol 50 (3).

Buss, D. M. (2002). "Review: Human Mate Guarding." Neuro Endocrinol Lett 23 (Suppl 4).

Blakemore SJ, Decety J (2001) From the perception of action to the understanding of intention. Nature Rev Neurosci 2: 561.

Buccino G, Vogt S, Ritzl A, Fink GR, Zilles K, Freund HJ, Rizzolatti G (2004) Neural circuits underlying imitation of hand actions: an event related fMRI study. Neuron 42: 323–34.

Caplan, A. (1992). Does the philosophy of medicine exist? Theoretical Medicine, 13, 67-77. http://dx.doi.org/10.1007/BF00489220

Cassell, E. J. (2004). The nature of suffering and the goals of medicine. New York: Oxford University Press. http://dx.doi.org/10.1093/acprof:oso/9780195156164.001.0001

Clifton-Soderstrom, M. (2003). Levinas and the patient as other: The ethical foundation of medicine. Journal of Medicine and Philosophy, 28, 4. http://dx.doi.org/10.1076/jmep.28.4.447.15969

Calder AJ, Keane J, Manes F, Antoun N, Young AW (2000) Impaired recognition and experience of disgust following brain injury. Nature Neurosci 3: 1077–1078.

Carey DP, Perrett DI, Oram MW (1997) Recognizing, understanding and reproducing actions. In: Jeannerod M, Grafman J (eds) Handbook of neuropsychology. Vol. 11: Action and cognition. Elsevier, Amsterdam.

Carr L, Iacoboni M, Dubeau MC, Mazziotta JC, Lenzi GL (2003) Neural mechanisms of empathy in humans: a relay from neural systems for imitation to limbic areas. Proc Natl Acad Sci USA 100: 5497–5502.

Changeux JP, Ricoeur P (1998) La nature et la règle. Odile Jacob, Paris.

Cochin S, Barthelemy C, Roux S, Martineau J (1999) Observation and execution of movement: similarities demonstrated by quantified electroencephalograpy. Eur J Neurosci 11: 1839– 1842.

Churchland, P.S. (1986), Neurophilosophy (Cambridge, MA: The MIT Press).

Churchland, P.S. & Ramachandran, V.S. (1993), 'Filling in: Why Dennett is wrong', in Dennett and His Critics: Demystifying Mind, ed. B. Dahlbom (Oxford: Blackwell Scientific Press).

Churchland, P.S., Ramachandran, V.S. & Sejnowski, T.J. (1994), 'A critique of pure vision', in Large- scale Neuronal Theories of the Brain, ed. C. Koch & J.L. Davis (Cambridge, MA: The MIT Press).

Crick, F. (1994), The Astonishing Hypothesis: The Scientific Search for the Soul (New York: Simon and Schuster).

Crick, F. (1996), 'Visual perception: rivalry and consciousness', Nature, 379.

Crick, F. & Koch, C. (1992), 'The problem of consciousness', Scientific American, 267.

Craig AD (2002) How do you feel? Interoception: the sense of the physiological condition of the body. Nature Rev Neurosci 3: 655–666.

Descartes, R. (1968). Discourse on method and meditations. Translated by F. E. Sutcliffe. New York: Penguin Books.

Descartes, R. (1998) Treatise on man. In S. Gaukroger (Ed.), The world

and other writings. Cambridge: Cambridge University Press. http://dx.doi.org/10.1017/CBO9780511605727.008

Dowrick, C. (1999). Uncertainty and responsibility. In C. Dowrick, & L. Frith (Eds.), General practice and ethics: Uncertainty and responsibility. London: Routledge.

Dworkin, G. (1988). The theory and practice of autonomy. Cambridge: Cambridge University Press. http://dx.doi.org/10.1017/CBO9780511625206

Damasio, A (2003a) Looking for Spinoza. Harcourt Inc. Damasio A

(2003b) Feeling of emotion and the self. Ann NY Acad Sci 1001: 253–261.

d'Aquili, Eugene. "Senses of Reality in Science and Religion." Zygon 17, no 4 (1982)

d'Aquili, Eugene. "The Biopsychological Determinants of Religious Ritual Behavior." Zygon 10, no. 1 (1975)

d'Aquili, Eugene. "The Myth-Ritual Complex: A Biogenetic Structural Analysis." Zygon 18, no. 3 (1983)

d'Aquili, Eugene, and Andrew Newberg. The Mystical Mind: Probing the Biology of Religious Experience. Minneapolis: Fortress Press, 1999.

Daly DD. 1958. Ictal affect. Am J Psychiatry.

Damasio, A. (1994) Descartes' Error: Emotion, Reason and the Human Brain. New York, Putnams.

Damasio, A. (1999) The Feeling of What Happens: Body, Emotion and the Making of Consciousness. London, Heinemann.

Darwin, C. (1859) On the Origin of Species by Means of Natural Selection. London, Murray.

Darwin, C. (1871) The Descent of Man and Selection in Relation to Sex. London, John Murray.

Darwin, C. (1872) The Expression of the Emotions in Man and Animals. London, John Murray; also published 1965, Chicago, University of Chicago Press.

Dawkins, M.S. (1987) Minding and mattering. In C. Blakemore and S. Greenfield (eds) Mindwaves. Oxford, Blackwell, 151-60.

Dawkins, R. (1976) The Selfish Gene. Oxford, Oxford University Press; a new edition, with additional material, was published in 1989.

Dawkins, R. (1986) The Blind Watchmaker. London, Longman.

Di Pellegrino G, Fadiga L, Fogassi L, Gallese V, Rizzolatti G (1992) Understanding motor events: A neurophysiological study. Exp Brain Res 91: 176–80.

Deikman, A.J. (2000) A functional approach to mysticism. Journal of Consciousness Studies 7(11-12), 75-91.

Delmonte, M.M. (1987) Personality and meditation. In M. West (ed.) The Psychology of Meditation. Oxford, Clarendon Press, 118-32.

Dennett, D.C. (1976) Are dreams experiences? Philosophical Review 73, 151-71; also reprinted in D.C. Dennett (1978) Brainstorms: Philosophical Essays on Mind and Psychology. Harmondsworth, Penguin, 129-48.

Dennett, D.C. (1987) The Intentional Stance. Cambridge, MA, MIT Press.

Dennett, D.C. (1988) Quining qualia. In A.J. Marcel and E. Bisiach (eds) Consciousness in Contemporary Science. Oxford, Oxford University Press, 42-77.

Dennett, D.C. (1991) Consciousness Explained. Boston, MA, and London, Little, Brown and Co.

Dennett, D.C. (1995a) Darwin's Dangerous Idea. London, Penguin.

Dennett, D.C. (1995b) The unimagined preposterousness of zombies. Journal of Consciousness Studies 2(4), 322-6.

Dennett, D.C. (1995c) Cog: steps towards consciousness in robots. In T. Metzinger (ed.) Conscious Experience. Thorverton, Devon, Imprint Academic, 471-87.

Dennett, D.C. (1995d) The path not taken. Behavioral and Brain Sciences 18, 252-3; commentary on N. Block, On a confusion about a function of consciousness. Behavioral and Brain Sciences 18, 227.

Dennett, D.C. (1996a) Facing backwards on the problem of consciousness. Journal of Consciousness Studies 3(1), 4-6.

Dennett, D.C. (1996b) Kinds of Minds: Towards an Understanding of Consciousness. London, Weidenfeld & Nicolson.

Dennett, D.C. (1997) An exchange with Daniel Dennett. In J. Searle (ed.) The Mystery of Consciousness. New York, New York Review of Books, 115-19.

Dennett, D.C. (1998) The myth of double transduction. In S.R. Hameroff, A.W. Kaszniak and A. C. Scott (eds) Toward a Science of Consciousness: The Second Tucson Discussions and Debates. Cambridge, MA, MIT Press, 97-107.

Dennett, D.C. (1998b) Brainchildren: Essays on Designing Minds. Cambridge, MA, MIT Press.

Dennett, D.C. (2001) The fantasy of first person science. Debate with D. Chalmers, Northwestern University, Evanston, IL, February 2001.

Dennett, D.C. (2003) Freedom Evolves. New York, Penguin.

Dennett, D.C. and Kinsbourne, M. (1992) Time and the observer: the where and when of consciousness in the brain. Behavioral and Brain Sciences 15, 183-247, including commentaries and authors' responses.

Dewhurst, Kenneth, and A. W. Beard. "Sudden Religious Conversions in Temporal Lobe Epilepsy." British Journal of Psychiatry 117 (1970)

Dewhurst K, Beard AW. Sudden religious conversions in temporal lobe epilepsy. 1970 Epilepsy Behav 2003

Devinsky O, Lai G. Spirituality and religion in epilepsy. Epilepsy Behav 2008.

Devinsky, O., Morrell, MJ, Vogt, BA. (1995) 'Contribution of anterior cingulate cortex to behavior', Brain, 118.

Eckhart Meister, Selected Writings

Fadiga L, Fogassi L, Pavesi G, Rizzolatti G (1995) Motor facilitation during action observation: a magnetic stimulation study. J Neurophysiol 73: 2608–2611.

Fogassi L, Gallese V, Fadiga L, Rizzolatti G (1998) Neurons responding to the sight of goal directed hand/arm actions in the parietal area PF (7b) of the macaque monkey. Soc Neurosci Abs 24:257.5.

Frith U, Frith CD (2003) Development and neurophysiology of mentalizing. Philos Trans R Soc Lond B Biol Sci 358: 459.

Frontera JG (1956) Some results obtained by electrical stimulation of the cortex of the island of Reil in the brain of the monkey (Macaca mulatta). J Comp Neurol 105: 365–394.

Farah, M.J. (1989), 'The neural basis of mental imagery', Trends in Neurosciences, 10.

Finlay BL, Darlington RB (1995) Linked regularities in the development and evolution of mammalian brains. Science 268.

Freud, S. "The Interpretation of Dreams", 1900

Freud, S. "Selected papers on hysteria and other psychoneuroses" Journal of Nervous and Mental Disease 1909.

Freud, S. "The Origin and Development of Psychoanalysis", 1910

Freud, S. "Psychopathology of everyday life", 1914

Freud, S. "Beyond the Pleasure Principle", 1920

Frith, C.D. & Dolan, R.J. (1997), 'Abnormal beliefs: Delusions and memory', Paper presented at the May, 1997, Harvard Conference on Memory and Belief.

Gay, Volney, ed. Neuroscience and Religion. Plymouth, UK: Lexington Books, 2009.

Gazzaniga, M. S. (1985). The social brain. New York: Basic Books.

Gazzaniga, M.S. (1993), 'Brain mechanisms and conscious experience', Ciba Foundation Symposium, 174.

Geschwind N. "Behavioural changes in temporal lobe epilepsy". Psychol Med. 1979.

Gellhorn, E., Kiely, W.F. "Mystical states of consciousness: neurophysiological and clinical aspects." J Nerv Ment Dis. 1972;154:399-405.

Gilbert SL, Dobyns WB, Lahn BT (2005) Genetic links between brain development and brain evolution. Nat Rev Genet 6.

Gray JA. The Psychology of Fear and Stress. 2nd ed. New York, NY: Cambridge University Press; 1988.

Gray JA. The Neuropsychology of Anxiety: An Enquiry into the Functions of the Septo Hippocampal System. 2nd ed. New York, NY: Oxford University Press; 2003.

Gloor, P. (1992), 'Amygdala and temporal lobe epilepsy', in The Amygdala: Neurobiological Aspects of Emotion, Memory and Mental Dysfunction, ed J.P. Aggleton (New York: Wiley-Liss).

Greenspan, S. I. and S. G. Shanker (2004). The first idea: How symbols, language, and intelligence evolved from our early primate ancestors to modern humans. Cambridge, MA: Da Capo Press.

Grady, D. (1993), 'The vision thing: Mainly in the brain', Discover, June.

Graham DT. Prediction of fainting in blood donors. Circulation. 1961;23:901-906.

Grubb BP, Olshansky B. Syncope: Mechanisms and Management. 1st ed. New York, NY: Futura Publishing Company; 1998.

Gallagher HL, Frith CD (2003) Functional imaging of 'theory of mind'. Trends Cogn Sci 7: 77.

Gallese V, Fogassi L, Fadiga L, Rizzolatti G (2002) Action representation and the inferior parietal lobule. In: Prinz W, Hommel B (eds) Attention & Performance XIX. Common mechanisms in perception and action. Oxford University Press, Oxford.

Gallese V, Keysers C, Rizzolatti G (2004) A unifying view of the basis of social cognition. Trends Cogn Sci 8: 396–403.

Gangitano M, Mottaghy FM, Pascual-Leone A (2001) Phase specific modulation of cortical motor output during movement observation. NeuroReport 12: 1489–1492.

Gangitano M, Mottaghy FM, Pascual-Leone A (2004) Modulation of premotor mirror neuron activity during observation of unpredictable grasping movements. Eur J Neurosci 20: 2193–2202.

Goldman AI, Sripada CS (2004) Simulationist models of face-based emotion recognition. Cognition 94: 193–213.

Grafton ST, Arbib MA, Fadiga L, Rizzolatti G (1996) Localization of grasp representations in humans by PET: 2. Observation compared with imagination. Exp Brain Res 112: 103–111.

Grèzes J, Costes N, Decety J (1998) Top-down effect of strategy on the perception of human biological motion: a PET investigation. Cogn Neuropsychol 15: 553–582.

Grèzes J, Armony JL, Rowe J, Passingham RE (2003) Activations related to "mirror" and "canonical" neurones in the human brain: an fMRI study. Neuroimage 18: 928–937.

Gross CG, Rocha-Miranda CE, Bender DB (1972) Visual properties of neurons in the inferotemporal cortex of the macaque. J Neurophysiol 35: 96–111.

Hippocrates. Hippocratic Corpus

Hari R, Forss N, Avikainen S, Kirveskari S, Salenius S, Rizzolatti G (1998) Activation of human primary motor cortex during action observation: a neuromagnetic study.

Proc. Natl Acad Sci USA 95: 15061–15065.

Hall, Daniel, Keith Meador, and Harold Koenig. "Measuring Religiousness in Health Research: Review and Critique." Journal of Religion and Health 47, no. 2 (2008)

Harris, Sam, Jonas Kaplan, Ashley Curiel, Susan Bookheimer, Marco Iacoboni, and Mark Cohen. "The Neural Correlates of Religious and Nonreligious Belief." PLoS One 4, no. 10 (October 1, 2009)

Halgren, E. (1992), 'Emotional neurophysiology of the amygdala within the context of human cognition', in The Amygdala: Neurobiological Aspects of Emotion, Memory and Mental Dysfunction, ed J.P. Aggleton (New York: Wiley-Liss).

Halligan PW, Fink GR, Marshal JC, Vallar G. 2003. Spatial cognition:

evidence from visual neglect. Trends Cogn Sci.

Handbook of Emotions, Edited by Michael Lewis, Jeannette M. Haviland-Jones, and Lisa Feldman Barrett, The Guilford Press; 3rd edition (2010).

Haggard, P., Clark, S. and Kalogeras, J. (2002) Voluntary action and conscious awareness, Nature Neuroscience 5, 382-5. Haggard, P., Newman, C. and Magno, E. (1999) On the perceived time of voluntary actions. British Journal of Psychology 90, 291-303.

Hameroff, S.R. and Penrose, R. (1996) Conscious events as orchestrated space-time selections. Journal of Consciousness Studies 3(1), 36-53; also reprinted in J. Shear (ed.) (1997) Explaining Consciousness-The Hard Problem. Cambridge, MA, MIT Press, 177-95.

Hardcastle, V.G. (2000) How to understand theN in NCC. InT.

Metzinger (ed.) Neural Correlates of Consciousness. Cambridge, MA, MIT Press, 259-64.

Harding, D.E. (1961) On Having no Head: Zen and the Re-Discovery of the Obvious. London, Buddhist Society.

Hardy, A. (1979) The Spiritual Nature of Man: A Study of Contemporary Religious Experience. Oxford, Clarendon Press.

Hamad, S. (1990) The symbol grounding problem. Physica D 42, 335-46.

Hamad, S. (2001) No easy way out. The Sciences 41(2), 36-42.

Harre, R. and Gillett, G. (1994) The Discursive Mind. Thousand Oaks, CA, Sage.

Haugeland, J. (ed.) (1997) Mind Design II: Philosophy, Psychology, Artificial Intelligence. Cambridge, MA, MIT Press.

Hauser, M.D. (2000) Wild Minds: What Animals Really Think. New York, Henry Holt and Co.; London, Penguin.

Hearne, K. (1990) The Dream Machine. Northants, Aquarian.

Hebb, D.O. (1949) The Organization of Behavior. New York, Wiley.

Helmholtz, H.L.F. von (1856-67) Treatise on Physiological Optics.

Heyes, C.M. (1998) Theory of mind in nonhuman primates. Behavioral and Brain Sciences 21, 101-48; with commentaries.

Heyes, C.M. and Galef, B.G. (eds) (1996) Social Learning in Animals: The Roots of Culture. San Diego, CA, Academic Press.

Hilgard, E.R. (1986) Divided Consciousness: Multiple Controls in Human Thought and Action. New York, Wiley.

Hodgson, R. (1891) A case of double consciousness. Proceedings of the Society for Psychical Research 7, 221-58.

Hofstadter, D.R. (1979) Code!, Escher, Bach: An Eternal Golden Braid. London, Penguin.

Hofstadter, D.R. and Dennett, D.C. (eds) (1981) The Mind's I: Fantasies and Reflections on Self and Soul. London, Penguin.

Holland, J. (ed.) (2001) Ecstasy: The Complete Guide: A Comprehensive Look at the Risks and Benefits of MDMA. Rochester, VT, Park Street Press.

Holmes, D.S. (1987) The influence of meditation versus rest on physiological arousal. In M. West (ed.) The Psychology of Meditation. Oxford, Clarendon Press, 81-103.

Holt, J. (1999) Blindsight in debates about qualia. Journal of Consciousness Studies 6(5), 54-71.

Horgan, J. (1994), 'Can science explain consciousness?', Scientific American, 271.

Holloway RL (1996) Evolution of the human brain. In: Lock A, Peters CR (eds) Handbook of human symbolic evolution. Oxford University Press, Oxford

Iacoboni M, Woods RP, Brass M, Bekkering H, Mazziotta JC, Rizzolatti G (1999) Cortical mechanisms of human imitation. Science 286: 2526–2528.

Iacoboni M, Koski LM, Brass M, Bekkering H, Woods RP, Dubeau MC, Mazziotta JC, Rizzolatti G (2001) Reafferent copies of imitated actions in the right superior temporal cortex. Proc Natl Acad Sci USA 98: 13995–13999.

Jeannerod M (1988) The neural and behavioural organization of goal-directed movements. Clarendon Press, Oxford.

Johnson-Frey SH, Maloof FR, Newman-Norlund R, Farrer C, Inati S, Grafton ST (2003) Actions or hand-objects interactions? Human inferior frontal cortex and action observation. Neuron 39: 1053–1058.

Jackson, F. (1982) Epiphenomenal qualia. Philosophical Quarterly 32, 127-36.

James, W. (1890) The Principles of Psychology (2 volumes). London, Macmillan.

James, W. (1902) The Varieties of Religious Experience: A Study in Human Nature. New York and London, Longmans, Green and Co.

Jansen, K. (2001) Ketamine: Dreams and Realities. Sarasota, FL,

Multidisciplinary Association for Psychedelic Studies.

Jay, M. (ed.) (1999) Artificial Paradises: A Drugs Reader. London, Penguin.

Jaynes, J. (1976) The Origin of Consciousness in the Breakdown of the Bicameral Mind. New York, Houghton Mifflin.

Johnson, M.K. and Raye, C.L. (1981) Reality monitoring. Psychological Review 88, 67-85.

Julien, R.M. (2001) A Primer of Drug Action: A Concise, Nontechnical Guide to the Actions, Uses, and Side Effects of Psychoactive Drugs (revised edn). New York, Henry Holt.

Kaada BR, Pribram KH, Epstein JA (1949) Respiratory and vascular responses in monkeys from temporal pole, insula, orbital surface and cingulate gyrus: a preliminary report. J Neurophysiol 12: 347–356.

Kohler E, Keysers C, Umiltà MA, Fogassi L, Gallese V, Rizzolatti G (2002). Hearing sounds, understanding actions: action Rrepresentation in mirror neurons. Science 297: 846–848.

Koski L, Wohlschlager A, Bekkering H, Woods RP, Dubeau MC (2002) Modulation of motor and premotor activity during imitation of target-directed actions. Cereb Cortex 12: 847–855.

Koski L, Iacoboni M, Dubeau MC, Woods RP, Mazziotta JC (2003) Modulation of cortical activity during different imitative behaviors. J Neurophysiol 89: 460–471.

Krolak-Salmon P, Henaff MA, Isnard J, Tallon-Baudry C, Guenot M, Vighetto A, Bertrand O, Mauguiere F (2003) An attention modulated response to disgust in human ventral anterior insula. Ann Neurol 53: 446–453.

Kandel, E. R. In Search of Memory: The Emergence of a New Science of Mind, W. W. Norton & Company (2007).

Kandel E. R. Schwartz JH, Jessel TM. Principles of neural sciences. New York; McGraw Hill, 2000.

Kanizsa, G. (1979), Organization In Vision (New York: Praeger).

Kaloupek DG, Scott JR, Khatami V. Assessment of coping strategies associated with syncope in blood donors. J Psychosom Res. 1985;29:207-214.

Kanwisher, N. (2001) Neural events and perceptual awareness. Cognition 79, 89-113; also reprinted inS. Dehaene (ed.) The Cognitive Neuroscience of Consciousness. Cambridge, MA, MIT Press, 89-113.

Kapleau, Roshi P. (1980) The Three Pillars of Zen: Teaching, Practice, and

Enlightenment (revised edn). New York, Doubleday.

Karn, K. and Hayhoe, M. (2000) Memory representations guide targeting eye movements in a natural task. Visual Cognition 7, 673-703.

Kasamatsu, A. and Hirai, T. (1966) An electroencephalographic study on the Zen meditation (zazen). Folia Psychiatrica et Neurologica Japonica 20, 315-36.

Kaiserman-Abramof, I. R., Graybiel, A. M., & Nauta, W. J. (1980). The thalamic projection to cortical area 17 in a congenitally anophthalmic mouse strain. Neuroscience, 5, 41–52.

Kanold, P. O., Kara, P., Reid, R. C., & Shatz, C. J. (2003). Role of subplate neurons in functional maturation of visual cortical columns. Science, 301, 521–525.

Kennedy, H., & Dehay, C. (1988). Functional implications of the anatomical organization of the callosal projections of visual areas V1 and V2 in the macaque monkey. Behav. Brain Res., 29, 225–236.

Kennedy, H., & Dehay, C. (1993). Cortical specifi cation of mice and men. Cereb. Cortex, 3, 171–186.

Koketsu, D., Mikami, A., Miyamoto, Y., & Hisatsune, T. (2003). Nonrenewal of neurons in the cerebral neocortex of adult macaque monkeys. J. Neurosci., 23, 937–942.

Komuro, H., & Rakic, P. (1992). Selective role of N-type calcium channels in neuronal migration. Science, 257, 806–809.

Komuro, H., & Rakic, P. (1993). Modulation of neuronal migration by NMDA receptors. Science, 260, 95–97.

Komuro, H., & Rakic, P. (1996). Intracellular Ca2+ fl uctuations modulate the rate of neuronal migration. Neuron, 17, 275–285.

Kornack, D. R., & Rakic, P. (1995). Radial and horizontal deployment of clonally related cells in the primate neocortex: Relation- ship to distinct mitotic lineages. Neuron, 15, 311–321.

Kornack, D. R., & Rakic, P. (1999). Continuation of neurogenesis in the hippocampus of the adult macaque monkey. Proc. Natl. Acad. Sci. USA, 96, 5768–5773.

Kornack, D. R., & Rakic, P. (2001a). Cell proliferation without neurogenesis in adult primate neocortex. Science, 294, 2127–2130.

Kornack, D. R., & Rakic, P. (2001b). The generation, migration, and differentiation of olfactory neurons in the adult primate brain. Proc. Natl. Acad. Sci. USA, 98, 4752–4757.

Kostovic, I., & Molliver, D. E. (1974). A new interpretation of the laminar development of cerebral cortex: Synaptogenesis in different layers of neopalium in the human fetus. Anat. Rec., 178, 395.

Kostovic, I., & Rakic, P. (1980). Cytology and time of origin of interstitial neurons in the white matter in infant and adult human and monkey telencephalon. J. Neurocytol., 9, 219–242.

Kostovic, I., & Rakic, P. (1984). Development of prestriate visual projections in the monkey and human fetal cerebrum revealed by transient cholinesterase staining. J. Neurosci., 4, 25–42.

Kennett, J. (1972) Selling Water by the River. London, Allen & Unwin; also published by New York, Vintage.

Kentridge, R.W. and Heywood, C.A. (1999) The status of blindsight. Journal of Consciousness Studies 6(5), 3-11.

Kihlstrom, J.F. (1996) Perception without awareness of what is perceived, learning without awareness of what is learned. In M. Velmans (ed.) The Science of Consciousness. London, Routledge, 23-46.

Kluver, H. (1926) Mescal visions and eidetic vision. American Journal of Psychology 37, 502-15.

Kollerstrom, N. (1999) The path of Halley's comet, and Newton's late apprehension of the law of gravity. Annals of Science 56, 331-56.

Kosslyn, S.M. (1980) Image and Mind. Cambridge, MA, Harvard University Press.

Kosslyn, S.M. (1988) Aspects of a cognitive neuroscience of mental imagery. Science 240, 1621-6.

Kinsbourne, M. (1995), 'The intralaminar thalamic nucleii', Consciousness and Cognition, 4.

Kjaer, Troels, Camilla Bertelsen, Paola Piccini, David Brooks, Jorgen Alving, and Hans Lou. "Increased Dopamine

Tone during Meditation- Induced Change of Consciousness." Cognitive Brain Research 13, no. 2 (April 2002)

Kölmel HW. 1985. Complex visual hallucinations in the hemianopic field. J Neurol Neurosurg Psychiatry.

Koenig, Harold. "Research on Religion, Spirituality, and Mental Health: A Review." Canadian Journal of Psychiatry 54, no. 5 (May 2009)

Koenig, Harold, ed. Handbook of Religion and Mental Health. San Diego, CA: Academic Press, 1998

Kraepelin E. Psychiatry: A Textbook for Students and Physicians. New York, NY: Science History Publications; 1990.

Lauglin, Charles, John McManus, and Eugene d'Aquili. Brain, Symbol, and Experience. 2nd ed. New York: Columbia University Press, 1992

Lakoff, G. and M. Johnson (1999). Philosophy in the flesh. Basic Books: New York.

LeDoux, J. E. (1996). The emotional brain. New York: Simon & Schuster.

LeDoux, J.E. (1992), 'Emotion and the amygdala', in The Amygdala: Neurobiological Aspects of Emo- tion, Memory and Mental Dysfunction, ed J.P. Aggleton (New York: Wiley-Liss).

Levin, D.T. and Simons, D.J. (1997) Failure to detect changes to attended objects in motion pictures. Psychonomic Bulletin and Review 4, 501-6.

Levine,J. (1983) Materialism and qualia: the explanatory gap. Pacific Philosophical Quarterly 64, 354-61.

Levine,J. (2001) Purple Haze: The Puzzle of Consciousness. New York, Oxford University Press. Levine, S. (1979) A Gradual Awakening. New York, Doubleday.

Levinson, B.W. (1965) States of awareness during general anaesthesia. British Journal of Anaesthesia 37, 544-6.

Lewicki, P., Czyzewska, M. and Hoffman, H. (1987) Unconscious acquisition of complex procedural knowledge. Journal of Experimental Psychology: Learning, Memory and Cognition 13, 523-30.

Lewicki, P., Hill, T. and Bizot, E. (1988) Acquisition of procedural knowledge about a pattern of stimuli that cannot be articulated. Cognitive Psychology 20, 24-37.

Lewicki, P., Hill, T. and Czyzewska, M. (1992) Nonconscious acquisition of information. American Psychologist 47, 796-801.

Manthey S, Schubotz RI, von Cramon DY (2003). Premotor cortex in observing erroneous action: an fMRI study. Brain Res Cogn Brain Res 15: 296–307.

Mesulam MM, Mufson EJ (1982) Insula of the old world monkey. III: Efferent cortical output and comments on function. J Comp Neurol 212: 38–52.

Naskar, Abhijit. "What is Mind?", 2016

Naskar, Abhijit. "In Search of Divinity: Journey to The Kingdom of Conscience", 2016

Naskar, Abhijit. "Love, God & Neurons: Memoir of A Scientist who found himself by getting lost", 2016

Naskar, Abhijit. "Neurons of Jesus: Mind of A Teacher, Spouse & Thinker", 2017

Naskar, Abhijit. "Rowdy Buddha: The First Sapiens", 2017

Naskar, Abhijit. "The Education Decree", 2017

Naskar, Abhijit. "Principia Humanitas", 2017

Naskar, Abhijit. "We Are All Black: A Treatise on Racism", 2017

Naskar, Abhijit. "Wise Mating: A Treatise on Monogamy", 2017

Naskar, Abhijit. "Illusion of Religion: A Treatise on Religious Fundamentalism", 2017

Naskar, Abhijit. "I Am The Thread: My Mission", 2017

Naskar, Abhijit. "Morality Absolute", 2017

Newberg, Andrew, and Jeremy Iversen. "The Neural Basis of the Complex Mental Task of Meditation: Neurotransmitter and Neurochemical Considerations." Medical Hypotheses 61, no. 2 (2003).

Newberg, Andrew. "How God Changes Your Brain: An Introduction to Jewish Neurotheology", CCAR Journal: The Reform Jewish Quarterly, Winter 2016.

Newberg, Andrew, and Stephanie Newberg. "A Neuropsychological Perspective on Spiritual Development." In Handbook of Spiritual Development in Childhood and Adolescence, edited by Eugene Roehlkepartain, Pamela King, Linda Wagener, and Peter Benson. London: Sage Publications, Inc., 2005

Newberg, Andrew. "The Neurotheology Link An Intersection Between Spirituality and Health", Alternative and Complimentary Therapies, Vol 21 No 1, February 2015.

Newberg, Andrew, Nancy Wintering, Dharma Khalsa, Hannah Roggenkamp, and Mark Waldman. "Meditation Effects on Cognitive Function and Cerebral Blood Flow in Subjects with Memory Loss: A Preliminary Study." Journal of Alzheimer's Disease 20, no. 2 (2010)

Nash, M. (1995), 'Glimpses of the mind', Time.

Nesse RM. Proximate and evolutionary studies of anxiety, stress and depression: synergy at the interface. Neurosci Biobehav Rev. 1999;23:895-903.

Nishitani N, Hari R (2000) Temporal dynamics of cortical representation for action. Proc Natl Acad Sci USA 97: 913–918.

Nishitani N, Hari R (2002) Viewing lip forms: cortical dynamics. Neuron 36: 1211–1220.

O'Hara, K. and Scutt, T. (1996) There is no hard problem of consciousness. Journal of Consciousness Studies 3(4), 290-302, reprinted in J. Shear (ed.) (1997) Explaining Consciousness. Cambridge, MA, MIT Press, 69-82.

O'Regan, J.K. (1992) Solving the "real" mysteries of visual perception: the world as an outside memory. Canadian Journal of Psychology 46, 461-88.

O'Regan, J.K. and Noe, A. (2001) A sensorimotor account of vision and visual consciousness. Behavioral and Brain Sciences 24(5), 883-917.

O'Regan, J.K., Rensink, R.A. and Clark,].]. (1999) Change-blindness as a result of "mudsplashes." Nature 398, 34.

Ornstein, R.E. (1977) The Psychology of Consciousness (2nd edn). New York, Harcourt.

Ornstein, R.E. (1986) The Psychology of Consciousness (3rd edn). New York, Pehguin.

Ornstein, R.E. (1992) The Evolution of Consciousness. New York, Touchstone.

Penfield W, Faulk ME (1955) The insula: further observations on its function. Brain 78: 445– 470.

Penrose, R. (1994), Shadows of the Mind (Oxford: Oxford University Press).

Penrose, R. (1989), The Emperor's New Mind: Concerning Computers, Minds and The Laws of Physics (Oxford: Oxford University Press).

Persinger, "'I would kill in God's name' role of sex, weekly church attendance, report of a religious experience and limbic lability" Perceptual and Motor Skills 1997.

Persinger "Experimental simulation of the God experience" Neurotheology 2003.

Persinger, M. A. (1993b). Personality changes following brain injury as a grief response to the loss of sense of self: Phenomenological themes as indices of local lability and neurocognitive restructuring as psycho- therapy. Psychological Reports, 72

Persinger, Corradini, Clement, Keaney, et al "Neurotheology and its convergence with neuroquantology" NeuroQuantology 2010.

Persinger, Koren and St-Pierre "The electromagnetic induction of mystical and altered states within the laboratory" Journal of Consciousness Exploration and Research 2010.

Persinger "Case report: A prototypical spontaneous 'sensed presence' of a sentient being and concomitant electroencephalographic activity in the clinical laboratory" Neurocase 2008.

Persinger and Saroka "Potential production of Hughlings Jackson's "parasitic consciousness" by physiologically-patterned weak transcerebral magnetic fields: QEEG and source localization" Epilepsy & Behavior 28 (2013).

Persinger. "The neuropsychiatry of paranormal experiences". J Neuropsychiatry Clin Neurosci 2001.

Persinger. "Neuropsychological bases of god beliefs", New York: Praeger, 1987

Persinger. "Temporal lobe epileptic signs and correlative behaviors displayed by normal populations", Journal of General Psychology, 1986

Persinger "Experimental Facilitation of the Sensed Presence: Possible Intercalation between the Hemispheres Induced by Complex Magnetic Fields" Journal of Nervous and Mental Disease 2002.

Palmer J. 1978. The out-of-body experience: a psychological theory. Parapsychol Rev.

Page AC. Blood-injury phobia. Clinical Psychology Review. 1994;14:443-461.

Perry BD, Pollard R. Homeostasis, stress, trauma, and adaptation. A neurodevelopmental view of childhood trauma. Child Adolesc Psychiatr Clin N Am. 1998;7:33.

Paré, D. & Llinás, R. (1995), 'Conscious and preconscious processes as seen from the standpoint of sleep-waking cycle neurophysiology', Neuropsychologia, 33.

P. S. de Laplace. Essai Philosophique sur les Probabilites [1814], in Academy des Sciences, Oeuvres Complotes de Laplace, Vol. 7, Gauthier-Villars, Paris (1886).

Perrett DI, Harries MH, Bevan R, Thomas S, Benson PJ, Mistlin AJ, Chitty AJ, Hietanen JK, Ortega JE (1989) Frameworks of analysis for the neural representation of animate objects and actions. J Exp Bio 146: 87–113.

Phillips ML, Young AW, Senior C, Brammer M, Andrew C, Calder AJ, Bullmore ET, Perrett DI, Rowland D, Williams SC, Gray JA, David AS (1997) A specific neural substrate for perceiving facial expressions of disgust. Nature 389: 495–498.

Phillips ML, Young AW, Scott SK, Calder AJ, Andrew C, Giampietro V, Williams SC, Bullmore ET, Brammer M, Gray JA (1998) Neural responses to facial and vocal expressions of fear and disgust. Proc R Soc Lond B Biol Sci 265: 1809–1817.

Puce A, Perrett D (2003) Electrophysiological and brain imaging of biological motion. Philosoph Trans Royal Soc Lond, Series B, 358: 435–445.

Pellegrino, E. D., & Thomasma, D. C. (1981). A philosophical basis of medical practice. New York: Oxford University Press.

Pellegrino, E. D. (1998). What the philosophy of medicine is. Theoretical Medicine and Bioethics, 19, 315-336. http://dx.doi.org/10.1023/A:1009926629039

Potter, R. (1996). Cambridge illustrated history of medicine. Cambridge: Cambridge University Press.

Raney, L. (2013). Integrated care: Evolving role of psychiatry in an era of health care reform. Psychiatric Services, 64, 11. http://dx.doi.org/10.1176/appi.ps.201300311

Ravez, L., & Tilman-Cabiaux, C. (2011). La Medicine autrement! Pour une éthique de la Subjectivité Médical. Namur: Presse Universitaires de Namur.

Rawls, J. (1999). A theory of justice. Cambridge: Harvard University Press.

Riordan, H. (1976). A humanistic approach to medical practice.

Dialogue: A Kansas Journal of Health Concerns, 3, 4

Ramachandran VS. Behavioral and magnetoencephalographic correlates of plasticity in the adult human brain. Proc Natl Acad Sci USA 1993; 90: 10413–20.

Ramachandran VS. Phantom limbs, neglect syndromes, repressed memories, and Freudian psychology. Int Rev Neurobiol 1994; 37: 291–333.

Ramachandran VS. Plasticity and functional recovery in neurology. Clin Med 2005; 5: 368–73.

Ramachandran VS, Hirstein W. The perception of phantom limbs. The D. O. Hebb lecture. Brain 1998; 121: 1603–30.

Ramachandran VS, McGeoch PD, Williams L, Arcilla G. Rapid relief of thalamic pain syndrome induced by vestibular caloric stimulation. Neurocase 2007; 13: 185–8.

Ramachandran VS, Rogers-Ramachandran D, Cobb S. Touching the phantom limb. Nature 1995; 377: 489–90.

Ramachandran VS, Rogers-Ramachandran D. Phantom limbs and neural plasticity. Arch Neurol 2000; 57: 317–20.

Ramachandran VS, Rogers-Ramachandran D. It's all done with mirrors. Sci Am Mind 2007; 18: 16–9.

Ramachandran VS, Rogers-Ramachandran D. Sensations referred to a patient's phantom arm from another subjects intact arm: perceptual correlates of mirror neurons. Med Hypotheses 2008; 70: 1233–4.

Ramachandran VS, Rogers-Ramachandran D, Stewart M. Perceptual correlates of massive cortical reorganization. Science 1992; 258: 1159–60.

Rizzolatti G, Craighero L (2004) The mirror-neuron system. Annu Rev Neurosci 27: 169–192.

Rizzolatti G, Scandolara C, Matelli M, Gentilucci M (1981) Afferent properties of periarcuate neurons in macaque monkeys. I. Somatosensory responses. Behav Brain Res 2: 125–146.

Rizzolatti G, Fadiga L, Matelli M, Bettinardi V, Paulesu E, Perani D, Fazio F (1996) Localization of grasp representation in humans by PET: 1. Observation versus execution. Exp Brain Res 111: 246–252.

Rizzolatti G, Fogassi L, Gallese V (2001) Neurophysiological mechanisms underlying the understanding and imitation of action. Nature Rev Neurosci 2:661–670.

Rock I, Victor J. Vision and touch: an experimentally created conflict between the two senses. Science 1964; 143: 594–6.

Rose´n B, Lundborg G. Training with a mirror in rehabilitation of the hand. Scand J Plast Reconstr Surg Hand Surg 2005; 39: 104–8.

Royet JP, Plailly J, Delon-Martin C, Kareken DA, Segebarth C (2003) fMRI of emotional responses to odors: influence of hedonic valence and judgment, handedness, and gender. Neuroimage 20: 713–728.

Rozin R Haidt J and McCauley CR (2000) Disgust. In: Lewis M, Haviland-Jones JM (eds) Handbook of Emotion. 2nd Edition. Guilford Press, New York, pp 637–653.

Saxe R, Carey S, Kanwisher N (2004) Understanding other minds: linking developmental psychology and functional neuroimaging. Annu Rev Psychol 55: 87–124.

Schienle A, Stark R, Walter B, Blecker C, Ott U, Kirsch P, Sammer G, Vaitl D (2002) The insula is not specifically involved in disgust processing: an fMRI study. Neuroreport 13: 2023–2026.

Showers MJC, Lauer EW (1961) Somatovisceral motor patterns in the insula. J Comp Neurol 117: 107–115.

Singer T, Seymour B, O'Doherty J, Kaube H, Dolan RJ, Frith CD (2004) Empathy for pain involves the affective but not the sensory components of pain. Science 303: 1157–1162.

Small DM, Gregory MD, Mak YE, Gitelman D, Mesulam MM, Parrish T (2003) Dissociation of neural representation of intensity and affective valuation in human gustation Neuron 39: 701–711.

Smith A (1759) The theory of moral sentiments (ed. 1976). Clarendon Press, Oxford.

Sprengelmeyer R, Rausch M, Eysel UT, Przuntek H (1998) Neural structures associated with recognition of facial expressions of basic emotions Proc R Soc Lond B Biol Sci 265: 1927–1931.

Strafella AP, Paus T (2000) Modulation of cortical excitability during action observation: a transcranial magnetic stimulation study. NeuroReport 11: 2289–2292.

Tanaka K (1996) Inferotemporal cortex and object vision. Ann Rev Neurosci. 19: 109–140.

Tomasello M, Call J (1997) Primate cognition. Oxford University Press, Oxford.

Tremblay C, Robert M, Pascual-Leone A, Lepore F, Nguyen DK, Carmant L, Bouthillier A, Theoret H (2004) Action observation and execution: intracranial recordings in a human subject. Neurology. 63: 937–938.

Umilta MA, Kohler E, Gallese V, Fogassi L, Fadiga L, Keysers C, Rizzolatti G (2001) "I know what you are doing": a neurophysiological study. Neuron 32: 91–101.

Visalberghi E, Fragaszy D. (2002). Do monkeys ape? Ten years after. In: Dautenhahn K, Nehaniv C (eds) Imitation in animals and artifacts. MIT Press, Boston. Pp. 471–500

Wicker B, Keysers C, Plailly J, Royet JP, Gallese V, Rizzolatti G (2003) Both of us disgusted in my insula: the common neural basis of seeing and feeling disgust. Neuron 40: 655–664.

Yokochi H, Tanaka M, Kumashiro M, Iriki A (2003) Inferior parietal somatosensory neurons coding face-hand coordination in Japanese macaques. Somatosens Mot Res 20 : 115–125.

Zald DH, Pardo JV (2000) Functional neuroimaging of the olfactory system in humans. Int J Psychophysiol 36: 165–181.

Zald DH, Donndelinger MJ, Pardo JV (1998) Elucidating dynamic brain interactions with across-subjects correlational analyses of positron emission tomographic data: the functional connectivity of the amygdala and orbitofrontal cortex during olfactory tasks. J Cereb Blood Flow Metab 18: 896–905.

TIME TO SAVE MEDICINE

TIME TO SAVE MEDICINE

…

TIME TO SAVE MEDICINE

www.ingramcontent.com/pod-product-compliance
Lightning Source LLC
Chambersburg PA
CBHW020425220526
45464CB00002B/568